Your Poisoned Plate:

Why you are sick, fat and tired

Allan P. Frank, MD, MS

Acknowledgements

Thank you to those who helped make this book possible:

Editors and Reviewers: Phillip Cook, Kimberly Beyer, Donald Frank

Cover designer: Kathy Haug

Disclaimer: No book can take the place of regular care by a healthcare provider.

GLOSSARY OF TERMS

Conventional*:* Plants grown using commercially available pesticides, herbicides or fertilizers. Conventional food contains man-made chemicals. May be additionally prepared and processed with artificial substances.

Organic: Plants grown using only naturally-occurring pest deterrents, weed/fungus deterrents and fertilizers. May not be prepared or processed with artificial substances.

Free Range: Animals that graze for their food in a natural, presumably pesticide free, environment. Can also apply to wild life that is harvested by hunters in the woods.

Wild Caught: Fish and other aquatic life that graze for their food in their natural environment.

Caged: Animals not free-range —usually fowl and small mammals such as rabbits.

Drug: Anything taken into the body in any manner with the intent to modify the biochemical reactions within the body. Pharmaceuticals, herbal supplements, vitamins, and recreational substances, including alcohol are all drugs.

GMO: Genetically Modified Organism. This broad definition can include both natural genetic modification, such as natural cross-breeding and cross-pollination as well as synthetic modification of a specific gene. For the synthetic modification, GMSO (definition below) is the preferred name.

GSMO: Gene Specific Modified Organism. Any plant or animal with a specific man-made genetic splice to a specific gene or gene set. This does not occur in nature in plants and higher animals and can rarely occur in nature in bacteria and viruses when man-made substances, such as antibiotics, are put into the environment.

Homeopathic: A philosophy that the most effective medicine is an infinite dilution of the active substance. It contains a defendable philosophy of a unifying hypothesis for diagnosis but indefensible treatments. In science, homeopathic treatments are completely at odds with the laws of physics and thermodynamics and Van der Waal forces (weak subatomic attraction between uncharged matter - analogous to the pull of gravity). Homeopathy should *not* be confused with Holistic.

Holistic: A philosophy considering the entire body, and to some degree, the emotional and spiritual aspects as well, in a healing interaction designed to return the body to homeostasis. Science supports holistic treatments as logical.

Homeostasis: The state of biochemical balance or equilibrium within the body.

Microbiome: The collection of microorganisms in your body and on your skin that are symbiotic and essential for optimal health. By number, there should be more microorganisms in and on the body than the actual number of human cells.

Toxin: A substance with the primary effect of harming or killing a living organism.

Toxic: An effect on the body that is detrimental to body function. The effect can be mild and temporary or fatal.

Author's Note & Introduction:

"A man too busy to take care of his health is like a mechanic too busy to take care of his tools."
—Spanish Proverb

After my third 20 minute diatribe of the day waxing on about nutrition and health to yet another aging patient wondering why there isn't a pill to cure her every symptom, I noticed her eyes glazing over and I paused. She said, "Dr Frank, this is just too much information for me. You should write a book."

And so I have.

This book arises from a unique perspective — that of a U.S. educated physician with advanced training in biochemistry, nutrition, and population health with experience in the clinical and regulatory research for both U.S. and European drug manufacturers. Having worked in governmental public health, academic and pharmaceutical company settings helped round out my understanding health politics. As intuitive as health is to me now, I am concerned daily when I hear patients say "I don't understand —I haven't done anything different and my body is just falling apart." My patients are not unique. I have heard the same lament in all five states in which I have been licensed to practice medicine. I am certain we waste our health chasing money, then we waste our money trying to regain the health we need not have ever lost.

I understand the body as a complex biochemical machine. On the whole I understand it better now than any healthcare provider I've encountered in the past three decades — and yet can with humility say the complexity of this fascinating creation still astounds and amazes me. We are gifted with this living machine at birth. We can knowingly sabotage this machine and stop its function in 20 years, we can neglect this machine and allow degeneration over 40 years, or we can maintain and support this machine so that it functions well at 100. Most people choose the middle road yet cannot understand why they are getting fatter, slower, sicker and more fatigued despite taking the latest marketed food supplement or pharmaceutical.

It is the middle road "average" person this book can help. It is written at a level that any average person can understand key points. But it also contains footnote references if you are interested in learning more. The self-sabotage group will destroy themselves regardless and the centurions don't need me, which leaves about 95% of the population who are in a place to listen and benefit. I like a challenge, particularly when I know the reward will be your good health. You simply need to decide if your health is worth your time.

You Have But One Life — Rise Up And Live It.

Form Leads Function

"He that takes medicine and neglects diet, wastes the
skills of the physician."
—Chinese proverb

Our bodies function as both simply and unfortunately a
collection of chemical reactions. Billions of reactions
occur in your body daily, catalyzed by thousands of
enzymes[1,2]. Each reaction will either move you toward
degeneration or toward repair. If you force your body out
of normal homeostasis, out of its natural balance, then
every reaction is degenerative.

Both degeneration and repair are necessary components
for any living thing. The science of all matter, living or
otherwise, is that nothing can become more structured
without the equivalent amount of destruction from
something else. In the case of our bodies, we degenerate
matter (food) to grow new tissue or to repair damaged
tissue. Consumption of food should contain only three
items to be more useful than hurtful. Anything other
than these three items will destroy the body more than
nourish the body.

---

[1] www.chm.qml.ac.uk/iubmb/enzyme Nomenclature Committee of the
International Union of Biochemistry and Molecular Biology
[2] Frey PA, Hegeman AD. Enyzmatic Reaction Mechanisms. Oxford University
Press. New York. 2006.

The Body's Three Main Requirements:

1. Energy (Calories). Living bodies require energy to drive all biochemical reactions. We call these energy units calories, which is simply a measurement of *how much* energy our body can expect from a particular food. There are not good calories or bad calories. Calories do not tell us how FAST that energy will be generated. Thus 100 calories of sugar water or candy calories are available in minutes, while 100 calories of egg are available in hours.

The body cannot safely handle quick calories in excess.

If you consume energy faster than you use it, your body will store some as glycogen (sugar linked together), some as fat and some will simply burn you from the inside (we call this glycosylation). Energy that your body cannot control will destroy the tissues around it. This is simple physics — laws of thermodynamics — the math of the relationship between matter and energy. A common example you can see is sun exposure : a little bit warms you and helps your skin make vitamin D; more than that damages your tissues and your body responds by tanning to protect itself; even more sunlight bypasses your body's defenses completely and kills the tissue (sunburn), and enough sun can cause heatstroke and death. It's all the same energy — but getting too much at one time is destructive rather than helpful.

2. Macronutrients (protein, carbohydrates, fats). Most foods are a combination of these because all plants and animals are composed of protein, complex carbohydrates and fats. With some exceptions (called "essential" nutrients) the cellular components of your body can change some macronutrients into other macronutrients. For example, carbohydrates can be broken down and reformed into fat; fat can be turned into ketone bodies for fuel. Sugar can be branched into more complex carbohydrates for short-term storage (glycogen — a fuel you use between meals and while you sleep.) While the most calories are gained from an equivalent amount of fat or protein, the body burns a lot of energy reorganizing these compounds into what it needs.   Many weight-loss diets use this fact to make the body inefficient. If you only eat protein, you burn enormous amounts of calories turning the protein into glucose (sugar) and fat into ketone bodies (another energy source).

3. Micronutrients (enzyme cofactors, such as vitamins and minerals). These substances are necessary in tiny amounts to break down the macronutrients and help form new molecules. These new molecules (proteins, fats and carbohydrates) combine to form body structures. These micronutrients can both help and hinder. In too large an amount, micronutrients can be harmful or even deadly. The toxicity of micronutrients varies – while vitamin C (ascorbic acid) is relatively harmless at large

doses, similar doses of vitamin A can kill you. Your body will tolerate large doses of sodium (salt) but a similar dose of iron is fatal. Micronutrients do not follow the adage of "if a little is good, a lot is better" but rather "when a little is good, a lot is not." Nature provides micronutrients that our body can use in amounts that are safe. Concentrating those nutrients in supplements without proper biochemical guidance can have unwanted consequences, usually in the form of kidney and liver failure, which can be permanent and even fatal.

How does the human body manage billions of reactions?

"The part can never be well unless the whole is well." — Plato

The short answer – with enzymes. More specifically, with enzymes that have been selected for superiority and survival by the natural environment over many thousands of years to give us health and reproductive advantage — but only within our ancestor's environment. Each cell has the potential for at least 30, 000 chemical reactions controlled by enzymes.

Imagine a factory assembly line that, rather than adding pieces one-by-one, added 30,000 pieces all at once and did this repeatedly. Man has created nothing close to this single cell. The closest example of a living cell would be a supercomputer, except that a supercomputer can only process energy while a living cell processes both energy and large molecules. Now imagine billions of factories processing 30,000 pieces AND coordinating with each other factory to ensure optimal efficiency. *That* is the human body. The body is as complex and wondrous as if every grain of sand at the beach was a supercomputer that never froze or crashed.

Unlike computers, living organisms have the good fortune of not needing a brain to direct every action. Unfortunately, to change any reaction within the body we cannot simply be reprogrammed with a few key strokes. The body is designed to function holistically, each part balancing with another redundantly so that if one part weakens, the body can survive while strengthening or circumventing the weakened function. The body strives to sameness — upset any balance and the body will act to restore the balance.

This balance is called *homeostasis*. The failure of homeostasis is the basis for most chronic disease; most failures in homeostasis occur when humans sabotage their own bodies, purposefully or not.

Human ancestors bequeathed to us, their progeny, a complex process requiring no active thought. Ancestors provided two functions necessary for continuation of their species: reproduction and the ability to catalyze (control and enhance) chemical reactions. A typical human cell has the ability to make over 30,000 proteins, many of these are enzymes. This ability preserves the life force in all cells and allows each cell to contribute something to the survival of other cells.

For cells to be effective, the body divides functions by tissues and organ systems. Organ systems are collections of similarly-minded tissues, tissues are groups of the same cell type. This division of labor means not all cells need do all things.

Cells specialize.

When the body begins at conception, the cells can potentially do anything but actually do very little. There is too much information in our genetic heritage for one cell to carry out all the instructions. These cells (for simplicity I will call them stem cells) carry all the information every cell in the body will ever need. These stem cells also know where to find the right information for each cell type.

A stem cell is like a librarian in a massive library containing all past information and future direction and has separated that information into areas by similar function, can tell you where to find a type of information, and what areas to avoid as useless in your information quest.

(A cancer cell, in contrast, is like a librarian Nazi socialist on acid in charge of the internet.)

When special functions are needed, the librarian gives the cell only that material needed, for example, "striated muscle", "retina", "hair follicle" or "pancreatic islet cell" and archives all the other unrelated information. The cell then becomes a specialist in that one topic and gathers with other specialists in that one topic. They unionize into a *tissue* to work together under identical rules and output then form an *organ*ization of similar functions, like a department, to increase their efficiency. The organization output is controlled by the organization, but the product and product rate can change if the boss *hormones* direct it or if the external suppliers *food* modify the starting materials.

Yes, well, my students don't like my analogies either.

To change the reactions within the body, we can either reprogram the body permanently — by extinction of bodies without the desired traits, by reproducing the desired traits in future generations, or both. We can, with targeted medication or medical techniques, change programming at a cellular level with genetic modification which generally modifies the biochemical reaction for the lifetime of one body and is not passed down to offspring. We can target a subset of reactions by absorbing drugs or drug-like substances. We can modify relative rates of reactions by what we ingest and what body parts and pathways we use.

Humans have learned some of this by instinct. When an action has reactions, negative or positive, the link is learnable by the organism. The more neural pathways available for information conveyance, the faster the organism learns.

A historical example may be useful. The Olympics existed long before biochemistry textbooks: humans learned that physical prowess improved with repeated practice.

Ancient peoples did not know about sacrolemmal nourishment and protection of sarcomere fibers in muscle cells or how to maximize muscle fibers by saturating the creatinine pathways with supplements or the histology of fast-twitch versus slow-twitch muscles, use of aerobic and anaerobic energy pathways or the build-up of the end product lactic acid which is linked to the sore muscles afterward. They did not know about testosterone, estrogen, cortisone, insulin and growth hormone only that some people responded differently to the same physical challenges and the difference was greatest between adult genders[3]. They didn't know about oxygen but they did know that they needed to breathe more when they used their bodies. They didn't know about calories but they did know they ate more when they used their bodies. Despite this lack of modern knowledge, they successfully grew their muscles and athletic prowess because their body chemistry knew and functioned without any conscious effort. All the ancient peoples knew was that if they did a sequence of physical moves, it got easier as they got stronger and as they got stronger, they performed increasingly difficult tasks.

---

[3] Nelson DL, Cox DM, eds. Lehninger Principles of Biochemistry, 6th ed. Hormonal Regulation and Integration of Mammalian Metabolism. Ch 23. W.H. Freeman and Co. New York NY. 2013.

Ancient peoples did not need to know about the function of melanocytes or the wavelength of ultraviolet light that activated the melanocytes. They did see that gradual exposure to the sun darkened their skin and made them more able to tolerate additional sun without burning. They did not see the link decades later to skin cancer as it was too far removed from the exposure and they probably died of infection or trauma long before old age.

Ancient peoples did not know they had hundreds of genes to help them detect when something smells or tastes good, bad, neutral or like a mate. If it tasted good they ate it. If it tasted bad they didn't eat or they died when they ate it. If it smelled like a reproductive opportunity, they took it. They did not refrain from eating something good due to worry about getting fat. They did not eat something that burned their mouths because someone else did it. They did not tell themselves "here comes an excellent genetic donor, I shall ovulate now or step up my sperm production and exude the appropriate pheromones."

The body does all of those things without any conscious thought IF you ensure it has a normal amount of natural substrate from which to work. Some think of basic action/reactions as common sense. *The body doesn't work by common sense; the body works through ancient sense.* That ancient sense is driven by ancient genes with a resistant but not impervious redundancy of biochemical reactions which are intricately coordinated through enzymes with no conscious effort.

You do not have to understand the body's complexity to accept its complexity. Beware, however, from tampering with something so complex when you know so little. This warning is not simply for the average person but for all healthcare professionals as well.

Knowing this and knowing that you cannot change this in less than several thousand years, you can be unhealthy and waste decades of time and money on pills and supplements or you can live more like a hunter-gatherer because, like it or not, living that way is what every cell in your body expects.

"Abandon the urge to simplify everything, to look for formulas and easy answers, and to begin to think multidimensionally, to glory in the mystery and paradoxes of life, not to be dismayed by the multitude of causes and consequences that are inherent in each experience -- to appreciate the fact that life is complex."
— M. Scott Peck

GSMOs: What you don't know CAN hurt you

"Once a rumor's spread, the truth is just a thing of the past." —Olivia Newton-John

"The same is true of GMOs." —Dr. Frank

As with everything worth discussion, definitions are important. Yelling louder at someone in English is only effective if that listener has a hearing problem AND speaks English. Yet we have a habit in America of speaking louder and repeating the same phrases regardless of the audience and are frustrated at the lack of a new response. So it is with GSMOs.

Wait — don't you mean GMOs? Not exactly, so let's establish some common language. GMO is an acronym for **G**enetically **M**odified **O**rganism. Unfortunately it has recently become synonymous with genetically engineered food where a specific gene is spliced into the plant.

The important questions for any GMO process is WHAT is being modified, HOW it is being modified, CAN it affect me and WHERE else does it impact my environment. Presently, only the first question is being answered.

The first question is important because if the modification is to the organism's inherited genome (the deoxyribonucleic acid or "DNA" for nearly all organisms), then the change is permanent — all the offspring, plant or animal, will have a 50 – 100% chance of carrying that change depending upon where the change was copied into the parent.

Not all changes in genes are permanent. There are genes that are only expressed under certain conditions — sometimes due to external forces, sometimes due to internal forces, sometimes a combination of both. The most common combined effect example of this is simple pregnancy. An external force from the male parent permanently changes a female cell, resulting in a new genetic organism that has traits from both. Further, that new organism releases hormones. Those hormones cause inactive genes in the female to become active, which in turn elicits numerous other changes in the female body. Some of these changes are temporary; some of these changes are permanent.

This is a genetic modification that occurs in nature. For sake of argument, let us agree that this genetic modification occurring in nature is generally good as it allows all species to survive.

Are there natural genetic modifications that are neutral? Yes. If we take the above example — pregnancy — and apply it to a horse and a donkey, we get viable offspring that cannot reproduce. From a horse or donkey perspective, that is probably a neutral modification unless one breeds all horses only with donkeys and vice-versa, which would result in both species and the mule generation to become extinct.

Well that could never happen. Or could it?

Precisely that has happened in plants we call grains. (And in general, it is happening in many plants that enthusiasts are trying to save called "heirloom" plants. However, the background for the most intrusive GMOs in the world started about twelve thousand years ago when human beings began growing huge amounts of very few crops we call grains. Over time, this transition from hunter-gatherer — where we and every other living thing simply ate what was available in nature — forced the agricultural need for farmers who were only successful if they could produce increasingly abundant crops to feed increasingly more people.

This change did not occur in a lab at the behest of some giant corporation. This change occurred through trial and error. Farmers were able to gradually increase the yield of crops by combining similar grasses and grains. Some of these combinations produced genetically new plants with the additive DNA of both parents —each combination produces a completely new species and cannot result in either of the parent species again. Fortunately, this doesn't happen in animals the way it does in plants.

Thus, what you call "wheat" would not be recognized as "wheat" to your ancestors. By studying frozen or mummified stomach remains from historical catastrophes, we can determine that "wheat" from five thousand years ago had about fourteen chromosomes. Historians call this "einkorn." Einkorn was crossed with another grass producing Emmer, a grain with 28 chromosomes, which was crossed a couple thousand years later with genus Triticum producing a 42 chromosome grass/wheat. Thus every few thousand years, farmers introduce a change in the food supply that, if successful, feeds people more efficiently. This millennial-long process does not seem to adversely impact the health of the human population. A more detailed history can be found in *Wheat Belly* by Dr William Davis, MD.

However, as our knowledge of botanical science and genetics has grown, so has our hubris. Rather than simply combining botanical species, we began breeding out characteristics people found objectionable. As a result, we have species of "wheat" that are very high in gluten, have very short growing times and much less fiber — traits which if introduced gradually over two thousand years might have been acceptable. Make the same changes over a few decades and the adverse impact discussed in Dr. Davis's book occurs.

It seems rather counter-intuitive at first. Why is it that making huge changes to a plant — in essence creating a new plant — is less troublesome than breeding out some genes we find less palatable. A completely acceptable answer is that we don't know. However, in this age of human hubris offering an educated theory seems acceptable as well.

How is it that humans ate einkorn and emmer and later triticum with no problem but cannot handle gluten-enhanced 2015 wheat?

The Theory of Food Adaptation[4] is that humans who successfully experience two food species individually for many generations and then experience the combination of the two plant species and their progeny for many generations can incorporate this genetic modification into their environment successfully. (Successfully meaning the humans continue to live healthy propagating lives.) This theory, while historically sound, obviously cannot be realistically tested.

It is probable that while most humans absorbed this food change in their diet successfully, some individuals did not. For example, if the combined "wheat" produced new substances that neither parent plant produced, or produced a substance in a higher/lower quantity, it is

---

[4] This theory is first introduced to the public in this text.

probable that some humans got sick or died. If the human species increased (and it did) as a result of the natural genetic modification, then the change was successful even if a few humans died from, for example, new "wheat" allergy. Thus WHAT was being modified was the entire plant. HOW it was being modified was provided for in nature. And humans had many generations over which to acclimate to these historical food changes.

Enter "wheat" 2015. In one generation scientists modified wheat genetically in numerous ways. Humans are not benefitting from the changes — we are getting sick. If only the small percentage who appear unaffected by the "wheat" changes reproduced, then history would judge this botany experiment successful as well. But based upon the sick teenagers and young adults in my medical practice I am doubtful. The changes made to "wheat" were too much and/or too quick.

When I first started my weight management clinic, one morbidly obese man was so incensed at my explanation of his poor food choices that he brought his wheelchair-bound elderly mother in with him at the next visit. She was not quite so portly as her son, but still overweight. "Tell her what you told me, that she's been poisoning me since childhood with bread and pies." I explained that I can't do that: the food his mother prepared for him 60 years before doesn't exist. The flour she bought from a local mill doesn't exist so that while his wife is trying to please him with comfort food that *looks* like his mother's bread, it is not. His mother simply shrugged her shoulders and said "I think he eats too much of the wrong food." Mom was right.   And so was I.

Mom knew that her son was now eating from a poisoned plate. And Mom is not alone. The Centers for Disease Control states that eighty percent of medical conditions are caused by our poor health choices. Where else have we seen that eighty percent?   In Dr McCleary's book[5] : "About eighty percent of the food on shelves of supermarkets today didn't exist 100 years ago."

The reason why eighty percent of our food didn't exist brings us back to the intent of this chapter — GSMO "Gene –SPECIFIC Modified Organisms" — and why each artificial manipulation of our food is potentially at least as detrimental to humans as "wheat" 2015.

Let us take a hypothetical example so this book can actually reach you without getting caught up in litigation.

Let us say you are a farmer with extensive rice-paddy land and your wife has advanced knowledge in botany and

[5] Larry McCleary, Feed Your Brain, Lose Your Belly: Experience Dynamic Weight Loss with the Brain-Belly Connection. 2011. Greenleaf Book Group Press. Austin TX.

biology. She also has very expensive tastes so she wants you to make more money so she can buy One Magnificent Mile in Chicago and a seat for your son on the New York Stock Exchange. After conferring, you decide that if it weren't for the weeds killing off the rice, you could easily make this money. The problem is, the weed killer also kills the rice.

Your wife is not deterred, she splices a gene for weed-killer resistance into the rice and encourages you to spray the weed killer copiously and often. You do and your yield is up 400%. Your daughter, a patent lawyer married to a U.S. Senator, patents the gene so that anyone trying to grow normal rice is forced to either buy your new rice or prove that the patented gene does not exist in their crops. Now everyone has to pay you to grow any rice. You are hugely successful and begin repeating this process for other plant species.

What could go wrong? Rice production is up so much that the world no longer worries about starvation. A few holier-than-thou physicians write some books about it and a few hippie moms get their undies in a bunch over genetically engineering their kid's food supply, but other than that there is no major public outcry and no political foe that money cannot buy off.

Ten years later, the cancer and obesity rates rise.

Why? Since weed killer no longer kills crops, it is used copiously and frequently. It seeps into the water supply. It is so concentrated on conventional produce that only wealthy people buying organic food avoid it. Diabetes rates skyrocket – rice is so inexpensive that it is used in everything and even becomes a source of high fructose syrup, further spreading what was once trace amounts of toxins. The higher levels of weed killer also mimic some neurotransmitters in the brain, and the autism and attention deficit diagnoses are up 55%. The amphibians that lived in the rice paddies couldn't reproduce due to the high levels of weed killer, so the mosquito population increased and malaria rates climbed. The snakes also died, so the rat population increased and now the first cases of bubonic plague are being reported in centuries. Autoimmune and food allergy illnesses increase around the world, causing growth retardation in children and chronic pain in adults that finally, after being linked to a neurotransmitter interference in the brain is no longer being called fibromyalgia. Further investigation of the GSMO rice showed that because of the location of the insertion in the rice gene, a downstream gene sequence was disturbed producing a modification in a rice protein. That modified protein is thought to be the cause of the food allergy affecting children by increasing asthma attacks and celiac disease.

These are medical possibilities I created within three minutes of the hypothetical product resulting from one gene splice. From that, you might surmise that I am anti-GMO/GSMO. You would be wrong. Science isn't good or bad; it is what we do with science that can be problematic. I avoid GSMOs for my family simply because there is insufficient safety information. That doesn't mean a given GSMO isn't safe. It means we just don't know.

The mistake we make in all matters concerning health is thinking this: if we don't know something, it must be safe. The truth is this: if we don't know something, we have no idea whether is it safe or not. Not knowing if something is safe is no different than putting a gun to your head and pulling the trigger. It is perfectly safe unless there is a bullet in the chamber you don't know about.

Calls by physicians for safety data have gone unheeded[6]. Among the top 64 industrialized nations, only the U.S. does not require GMOs to be labeled. You have no way to know if your food is GMO or normal in the United States. History is unfolding in much the same manner as the "hypothetical" anecdote above: "Round-Up" (glyphosate) application is being used 250 times more than at inception and "2,4-D" (2,4-dichlorophenoxyacetic acid) is

---

[6] Landrigan PJ, Benbrook C. GMOs, Herbicides, and Public Health. N Engl J Med 2015. 373:8. 693-695.

about to launch as a combined product with Round-Up which will be liberally sprayed on your food[7]. If you don't know what 2,4- D is, for a non-chemist it is synonymous with Agent Orange. On and in your food.

A responsible people would require genetic modification be fully and transparently researched. Rollout should be limited until safety research is completed and publicly released. There should be NO patent protection for any genetic modification to a food or food product. That would allow farmers to produce non-modified products without ending up in court or incurring insurmountable legal defense costs. It would greatly reduce the rate of genetic food modification. No one should legally prevent you from purchasing unmodified food, but that is precisely the legal environment we now have. Finally, no one should have the power to inflict upon the world a basic food change. It is simply too vital a human need, and no company ever has had the resources to repair the damages that could be irrevocably done to the human food supply.

---

[7] Duke SO. Perspectives on transgenic herbicide-resistant crops in the United States almost 20 years after introduction. Pest Manag Sci 2015:71:652-657.

If you want more detailed background:

Scientists discovered in 1946 that DNA can transfer between organisms. The first genetically modified plant was produced in 1983, using antibiotic-resistant tobacco. In 1994, the transgenic Flavr Savr tomato was approved by the FDA for marketing in the US. The modification delayed ripening after picking.

In 1995, several transgenic crops received marketing approval: canola with modified oil composition (Calgene), *Bacillus thuringiensis* (Bt) corn/maize (Ciba-Geigy), cotton resistant to the herbicide bromoxynil (Calgene), Bt cotton (Monsanto), Bt potatoes (Monsanto), glyphosate-tolerant soybeans (Monsanto), virus-resistant squash (Monsanto-Asgrow), and additional delayed ripening tomatoes (DNAP, Zeneca/Peto, and Monsanto). In 2000, scientists genetically modified rice to increase its nutrient value. As of 2011, the United States is the leading country in the production of genetically-modified foods. As of 2013, roughly 85% of corn, 91% of soybeans, and 88% of cotton produced in the US are genetically modified.

Conventional Food – Killing me softly

"A Who's Who of pesticides is therefore of concern to us all. If we are going to live so intimately with these chemicals eating and drinking them, taking them into the very marrow of our bones – we had better know something about their nature and their power."

— Rachel Carson, *Silent Spring*

"A nation that destroys its soils destroys itself."

—Franklin D. Roosevelt

Organic unprocessed food is what our bodies are designed to eat. If that is all you wanted to know, skip to the end of the chapter. Otherwise hang on for some fun facts.

After World War II, we had a surplus of synthetic nitrogen and other chemicals that could no longer be used to kill the Nazis and Imperialists. The war had fostered an unparalleled growth in chemistry intellect and mass-production ability to meet that challenge. Nitrogen can be modified to either quickly release energy, resulting in an explosion, or slowly to incorporate into the food cycle in the soil. Realizing this, chemists provided an option to bombs: fertilizer. By enriching the soil with concentrated nitrate from factories, farmers need not rely on manure and crop rotation. Once farmers realized that enriched soil generated rapid plant growth, they were hooked. It seems that unlike animals, who simply get fat when we eat too much energy (food), plants grow big quickly.

The background follows in a textbox for readers who wish to have more detail.

Post World War II Agriculture

The Haber-Bosch method for synthesizing ammonium nitrate was a breakthrough allowing crop yield increase. It was first patented by German chemist Fritz Haber. In 1910 Carl Bosch, while working for German chemical company BASF, successfully commercialized the process and secured further patents. Following World War II, synthetic fertilizer use increased rapidly, keeping with the increasing world population.

The Green Revolution generally refers to post WWII through the 1970s when bioscience markedly increased agriculture production. Norman Borlaug is often cited as the "Father of the Green Revolution", credited globally for nearly eliminating starvation. This time period produced high-yielding cereal grains, irrigation expansion, technology modernization, distribution of hybridized seeds, synthetic fertilizers, and sadly, pesticides and other growth modulation techniques to farmers.

Synthetic nitrogen, pesticides and herbicides increased crop yields within a single generation in the 20th century. Overabundance of grain allowed for a shift from pasture-raised to grain-fed animals, subsequently reducing the cost of livestock. Further high-yield staple grains such as rice, wheat, and corn are continually reinvented through mainly synthetic means. The Green Revolution involved exporting not the product but also the technologies (pesticides, herbicides, synthetic fertilizers) of the developed world to the developing world. This short-sighted but understandable revolution thereby circumvented prior concern that Earth would be unable to support its population.

World War II brought other advances as well.

To save sick soldiers on both sides of the war, scientists bolstered medications first with the German-owned Bayer company's discovery of sulfa antibiotics (known as Prontosil) eventually leading to sulfa overuse in the United States and Europe. Because no patent protection was issued for the active substance sulfanilamide, anyone could use sulfa in any concoction with any claims. This unrestricted use resulted in the United State's first major adverse experience with food additives when many children (and some adults) were cured of their infections only to die slowly and painfully as a result of ingesting a health elixir containing a toxic additive diethylene glycol (now known most commonly as antifreeze).

The U.S. government reacted by forming the Federal Food, Drug and Cosmetic Act (FDA) in 1938, reducing the risk of future medical misadventures and ushering in an era of false security for Americans who previously lived by "caveat emptor" (beware buyer) and did not expect safety from everything they purchased. The public safety provision made by the U.S. government was understandable and in retrospect helpful in preventing future direct harms as discussed next. However, the change in philosophy — new complacency — by the U.S. consumer would soon become dangerous to their health.

In the 1950s Europe released thalidomide, a sedative and immune-system modulation medication now known to cause severe birth defects. Because U.S. federal law prohibited its sale in the United States, the thalidomide tragedy largely spared U.S. children and caused the U.S. Congress under John F. Kennedy's administration to strengthen federal protections — medications now had to pass clinical trials in humans. These clinical trials results had to obtain the U.S. FDA approval prior to selling medications in the United States. Falsely assuaging U.S. consumers, the US FDA would release drugs with a statement of "Safety and Efficacy," that actually describes only short-term side-effects and the medical response expected for the intended use of the medication. It does not mean the product is generally safe and effective in any absolute terms, but that hasn't stopped drug companies from marketing it directly to consumers nor has it stopped lawyers from financial windfalls for patients who make erroneous and sweeping safety assumptions far beyond the product's approval provisions.

Companies and consumers alike vilify the FDA. They should not. These are generally underpaid people (they work more hours than congressmen and have more education than most teachers) who feel strongly about protecting you. Rather than blame one of the few government agencies doing their job well, the U.S. consumer would be better protected by stopping direct-to-consumer advertising, including internet advertising. If the consumer wants to know the specifics about a drug, they can do what physicians do: read the FDA-approved package insert.

On the flip-side of the coin, well-meaning physician activists have shot the medical community in the foot by overly-restricting drug company access to physicians. While week-long cruises and baseball game box seats may be overly influential, giving a physician lunch, branded pens, notepads and plastic bags — yes plastic bags — hardly compromises our patient loyalty. Indeed, once the "gift" falls under about $300 it is not even worth the physician's time, suggesting that economically a physician would be biased AGAINST a drug company that offers an ink pen with a plastic bag for drug samples. Further, when Health Maintenance Organizations (HMOs – a type of health insurance company) studied financial influence needed to coerce physicians to change any practice that the physician felt might not be advantageous to their patient, they would have to pay the physician a bonus of at least 10% of their standard salary. Medical activists wrongly associate brand recognition with medical influence and have harmed continuing medical education as result. The two are not interchangeable.   But lest I digress further, back to organic food.

The false sense of security that Americans had for their medications soon extended to their food, protected under similar but far less stringent federal requirements. To understand the weakness of food (and cosmetic) protections, first understand that *every* weakness in the drug safety protection extends to food and food additives.

What are food additives? Pick up any prepackaged food. Look at the label. Everything listed on the label that you do not recognize is an additive. Anything that has a number associated with the name, such as "yellow dye #6" is an additive. *Anything* that you cannot see grown on a farm or swimming in a lake or ocean is a food additive. Food additives do not belong in your food. Food additives are not natural; your body abhors unnatural substances. Your body is not equipped to process food additives and must treat food additives as toxins. These food additives are the ones you knowingly ingest.

But are there toxic food additives that you don't know about?

Yes. Toxicity aside, the danger of food additives, pesticides and food-like substances is that there are few protective strengths in the law. Given laxity of food import laws internationally and across state lines, this is not surprising. Were food to be studied and labeled as extensively as medication, the regulatory cost would halt food production and we would actually have true hunger and starvation in America for the first time since the 1930s.

Regarding the organic food philosophy, know the FDA is prohibited from classifying the following as food additives: pesticides, pesticide residues, color additives and any substance grandfathered into law (in existence prior to 1958), drugs given to animals you eat, or chemicals intended for use as a dietary supplement. If the FDA cannot regulate it, they cannot force the manufacturer to warn you about it. These are equally concerning food additives: substances *in your food* that do not even appear on the food label.

The other allowable substances in your food are natural but not necessarily nutritious: maggots, insect parts, rodent hair, mold, fly eggs and mammal feces. The more the food is processed, the greater percentage of vermin substances is allowed. Educational, isn't it? While it disgusts our western culinary sensibilities, recall that in nature and in your own kitchen you are eating some of these things every day — probably more cockroach feces, insect parts and sloughed skin/hair of local mammals, pets and scavenging rodents alike.

If you give most Americans the choice between eating peanut butter with rat poop or peanut butter with pesticides, they will and do choose the latter. That is the wrong choice.

Humans have evolved over millennia to eat rat poop (within reason) and insect parts — but not pesticides. We can derive nutrition from maggots and other grubs but not from food additives. Humans can and do live from insect protein safely; humans can and do live from rodents safely.

For example, one of my grandfather's favorite dishes was smothered squirrel. My grandmother would open a second story window of their farmhouse and plug a couple squirrels with her .22, dress them and stick them in the oven. She died just shy of her 99th birthday. They had an organic farm back before "organic" was a catchphrase; we just all hated the way food tasted the one year they tried conventional fertilizer.

Why is this important? Because Americans wrongly assume that conventional or processed food is somehow cleaner. There is no legal reason for food to be less free of natural waste and insect bystanders whether or not it is packaged and processed. Logically, the more places food has to travel before reaching your poisoned plate, the more chance it has of natural contamination by insects and rodents foraging for food. More importantly, the more people process your food, the greater the contamination with human sweat, snot, saliva, blood and feces. It is the human contamination that is more dangerous to you. (Despite the law, no observant person visiting any common restroom can fail to see the number of patrons and employees who fail to wash their hands prior to leaving the restroom.)

Non-organic (and processed organic) food has at least as much likelihood as organic food of having natural insect and rodent waste. All processed food has a greater likelihood of having human waste. In short, conventional and processed food is not cleaner than organic or locally-purchased food.

That leaves us with one main difference: chemicals added to food during growth, harvest or processing. This one difference is the main reason to eat organic.

Organic food is not more nutritious. There are enough conflicting studies (one of my academic appointments is from Michigan State University – arguably the strongest agricultural research group in the nation, and there are skeptics on both sides of the argument) to reasonably conclude there isn't much difference in the *nutrition* of organic produce compared to conventional produce. In other words, the vitamins and macronutrients from organic produce and conventional produce is the same.

The reason to choose organic produce is for what it does *not* have: herbicides, pesticides and synthetic fertilizer residues. Similarly, organic animal products do not have added antibiotics, hormones or residue from eating food that has herbicides, pesticides and fertilizers. Unlike organic produce, there is growing evidence that wild or free-range animals are more nutritious than conventional farmed or grain-fed animals. Thus "organic" is not the only item of interest for animal products — ideally you want "grass-fed" or "free range" as well. The reason for this is, again, due to our ancient ancestors and how they evolved.

In the Paleolithic era, humans consumed essential fats (the omega-6 and omega-3 fat) in 1:1 ratio that we know naturally occurred in free-range meat, fish, plants, nuts and fruit.[8] In contrast, Americans consume over ten times the amount of omega-6 compared to omega-3, a pro-inflammatory ratio that our genetic heritage does not accommodate. The highest sources of omega-6 in our diet come from common oils: corn oil, soy oil, canola oil, safflower oil – which you will find in almost every

[8] Simonpoulos AP. Omega-3 fatty acids and antioxidants in edible wild plants, nuts and seeds Asia Pac journal of Clin Nutrition. 2002. Doi: 10.1111/ajc.2002.11.issue-s6/issuetoc.
Robinson F. Power-Packed Purslane. Mother Earth News. April/May 2005.
n-3 Fatty Acids in Eggs from Range-Fed Greek Chickens. N Engl J Med. 1989;321(20):1412-1412.
Van Vleit T, Katan MB. Lower ratio of n-3 to n-6 fatty acids in cultured than in wild fish. Am J Cin Nutr 1990.

condiment, dessert and processed baked good. We also get the inflammatory omega-6 oils in farm-raised animals (beef, pork, chickens and fish). While the common starting point of food is a farm, this can also be where processing occurs. Food that is grown in a non-natural way is processed, but we define that as "farm-raised" or "grain-finished" to make it sound healthier. It may be tastier, but it is not healthier.

Why are they called "omega -3" or "omega-6"? The naming of biochemical compounds follows convention. The textbox that follows provides more detail, but it is not critical to the discussion.

How fats and oils are named

Traditional biochemists would call the most common omega-3 fat "cis, cis, cis-9,12,15-Octadecatrienoic acid" and that is what they would expect a graduate student to give them on the test when given the structural formula $CH_3CH_2CH==CHCH_2CH==CHCH_2CH==CH(CH_2)_7COOH$. So that physicians wouldn't feel inadequate at cocktail parties, biochemists would use the term α-Linoleic acid. Omega-3 is a colloquialism of sorts, referring to the placement of a double-bond (==) at carbon #3 counting from the tail-end (omega) of the carbon skeleton. Food container labeling is simpler using the omega-3 terminology and it makes for much shorter articles in print as well.

To make this a bit easier to understand: Fatty acids are fats and oils. Fatty acids with the first double bond in the same place behave similarly in our body. For example, α-Linoleic acid and docosahexanenoic acid (DHA) are both "omega-3" oils, but when you buy fish oil as a supplement, it is the docosahexanenoic acid you are purchasing. When you buy various seed/nut oils, it is α-Linoleic acid, even though both are advertised as "omega-3."

For normal people to understand food labels about fat, the knowledge of saturated versus unsaturated is crucial. The presence of any double bond places the fat in the "unsaturated" category. When you read "polyunstaturated" (poly = many) the fat has more than one double bond (such as the omega-3 and omega-6 fats). Monounsaturated fats have only 1 (mono = one) double bond. Saturated fats have no double bonds.

The more double bonds, the lower the temperature at which the fat stays liquid. As a quick test, any oil you put in the refrigerator that stays liquid is unsaturated. When you read about "PUFAs," the reference is to **p**oly**u**nsaturated **f**atty **a**cids.

For example, the omega-6 to omega-3 ratio of wild caught salmon is 2.0, but the farmed salmon ratio is 6.1 — three times more inflammatory for the same fish simply raised on different food (nature versus farmed)! Eggs from free-range chickens are higher in healthful non-inflammatory fat than are eggs from caged chickens. Conventional milk has a ratio of 12.6, whereas organic milk ratio is 5.1. People are no different than cows in that respect; the ratio of inflammatory fats in breast milk is the same as the ratio of inflammatory fats in the mother's diet.

And why is inflammation bad you ask? Inflammation is not always bad. Inflammation is often helpful when it is initiated by the body to protect the body. Inflammation is a chemical response by the body when the tissues are damaged. The chemicals released swell the area to contain the damage and bring infection-fighting cells into the area. Inflammation causes pain because swelling causes pressure; pressure sensors in the body register this stimulus as pain. In amounts controlled by the body, inflammation protects and initiates healing.

But when too much inflammation occurs, blood and other body fluids do not flow normally. The immune system cells destroy normal tissue and tissue repair is inhibited. Excess blood clotting occurs. Swelling is prolonged and thus pain is prolonged. Inflammation is bad when it occurs in too much an amount over too long a period of time. For the body to control inflammation in a manner that is more helpful than harmful, the body must have a natural ratio of inflammatory to anti-inflammatory oils in the diet. The normal ratio that occurs in human diets in nature is between 1:1 and 2:1. When the diet contains the balance provided in unprocessed food, the body regains control of inflammation. The ratio in the average American diet is at least 12: 1, which eliminates the body's control in a way that greatly favors inflammatory damage instead of repair.

This is not top-secret information. American taxpayers have been ignoring the information they've paid for. The National Health Service has documented that mortality risk increases with each serving of grain-fed red meat and that risk of death increased more if the meat was processed. Common processed meat includes: hot dogs, sausage, salami, lunch meat and, yes, bacon. Physicians verify this: persons eating an average additional serving of grain-fed red meat, mortality risk increased by thirteen percent; for each serving of grain-fed processed meat, mortality risk increased by twenty percent[9]. A "serving" is three ounces – a little less than two hot dogs or three slices of bacon.

U.S. physicians have known for decades that diets high in processed foods, especially meats, result in more disease and shorter lives. But then doctors and nurses have known for seventy years that smoking did the same thing, and we smoked just like everyone else. Knowing a thing and acting logically are two distinct actions. Emotional choices drive most of our life choices. If emotion was not the main driver for illogical choices, all persons in the marketing business would be unemployed. Marketing is simply the art of manipulating people's emotions in a way that encourages them to purchase a product or service. Fortunately, we still live in a semi-free country where we can make unhealthy choices so there is plenty of money for persons convincing us to make purely emotional stupid choices.

---

[9] Sun Q. Read Meat Consumption and Mortality. Arch Intern Med 2012; 172(7):555.

What about unprocessed conventional meat? There is no such thing.

In the United States, healthy farm animals are given twenty-five million pounds of antibiotics every year. The reason is simple: farm animals given antibiotics get fat and consumers like meat with lots of fat. It is not possible to buy conventional meat that does not have man-made chemicals added. Some antibiotics are added directly into food or even injected into the animal; some are added indirectly through pesticides sprayed on the animal or around the farm environment and animal food. If antibiotics make otherwise healthy farm animals fat, a reasonable hypothesis is that antibiotics make otherwise healthy humans fat as well[10].

Before vilifying farmers for giving you what you demanded — obese animals for obese people — consider that nearly every household in America pushes antibiotics into public drinking water every day. We apply broad spectrum antibiotic ointments for every tiny scratch, completely without any need verbalized from a health care professional. We use antibiotic soaps inappropriately, washing antibiotics into our water supply where those same chemicals make harmful bacteria resistant to antibiotics. When we are actually in medical need of the antibiotics, these antibiotics are then

---

[10] Morgan KK. Are Antibiotics Making us Fat? Genome. Summer 2015. 42-49.

ineffective. Consider the long leash of irresponsibility we have given our own selves in our own homes before shortening the leash on farmers trying to make a living. Thus we have all contributed daily to processed, adulterated food and water.

If processed food is an unhealthy choice, what about organic unprocessed food?

Recall organic plants are those grown using only naturally-occurring pest deterrents, weed/fungus deterrents and fertilizers. Further, organic produce may not be prepared or processed with artificial substances. Processed food is any significant change in the form of the food from the natural state. It is important to understand the difference between minimally processed and extensively processed food. The more food is processed, the more poisonous it is to your body.

For example, fresh green beans from the produce section can be either organic or conventional, depending upon how the farmer grew the beans. The green beans in the grocery's produce section are unprocessed — the green beans are in their natural state. However, if you go to the freezer section of the store, you can find loose frozen green beans sliced up. Just like the fresh green beans, the frozen green beans can be either organic or conventional. Loose frozen green beans will say "green beans" on the label, that is all. These are minimally processed —

machine separated and cut but uncooked and with nothing added. Minimally processed foods are acceptable and still nutritious to your body. However, if you find "green bean casserole" in the freezer section, it is highly processed and toxic to your body. If you find green beans in the canned section, it is highly processed and toxic to your body. It is far better for your body to skip meals than it is to eat highly processed food. Never waste your money buying organic food *if it has been highly processed*.

So what would be the best food for your body?

Organic unprocessed food is what our bodies are designed to eat. Organic unprocessed food is what our ancient ancestors ate. Maximizing your body chemistry means purchasing organic unprocessed foods and learning to prepare organic unprocessed foods without using artificial chemicals. It also means learning how your food came to be your food or growing food yourself.

You don't know where that banana's been

"Our bodies are our gardens – our wills are our gardeners." —William Shakespeare (paraphrased)

"Do not call anything impure that God has made clean." —The Bible. Acts 10:15

After getting past the shock of "but what am I going to eat?!" from our first discussion about eliminating processed foods, the next shock by my patients occurs when discussing their current food choices. They show me an exhaustive list of (mostly) fresh produce. This is when the organic discussion happens.

I do not mandate my patients eat organic. I do not mandate my patients eat in any particular way whatsoever. I simply empower them to live the healthiest life they wish. In this I accede to the Shakespeare quote – it is the will of the patient that will largely determine the health of their body. I can and will step in when fate throws the patient a curve, but western medicine is notoriously poor at modifying health outcomes for chronic diseases. Most chronic diseases are maladies that occur from chronically improper nutrition.

Give us a traumatic event, a stopped heart, an infection or a blood clot and we are close to the gods we sometimes think ourselves. Give us diabetes, obesity, cancer and myriads of other problems and we will merely slow your drive to the morgue. Physicians say "treat" when they don't mean "cure." When you hear "treat" we are saying we cannot fix it. It's better than nothing, but frankly not what most physicians thought we were signing up for when walking into our first medical school lectures.

In medical school, we are generally taught to *do* something to the patient. Whether by knife, needle, pill or salve, we intervene. It is never politically correct to suggest that we can do very little for someone who persists in bad choices, nor are we paid to do so. The reimbursement by the government is the highest for cutting on the patient and either taking something out or putting something in, followed by the prices for infusing expensive chemicals into the patient, then by prescribing chemicals for them to ingest, and last — last on the list!— is counseling for behavior change which is generally not covered by insurance.

I frequently quip to my family that I should have been a proceduralist — an ophthalmologist can make more money in 15 minutes removing a cataract (something a robot can do) than I can make in an entire week trying to save a diabetic from losing a kidney and more than I can make in a month of counseling smokers to stop. This is not meant as a gripe. It simply demonstrates what

Americans value; we value techniques over knowledge. And we do not value time —at least not other peoples — at all.

With this backdrop, it is easier to understand why everyone doesn't get counseled to change their bad habits. No one pays for it. However, if we let you get sick, we can do things to you and make a lot more money. You'll get even sicker because we aren't curing you and we make even more money. I am not suggesting the physicians consciously think this way. This simply puts to words the incentive structure you've given to physicians.

Yet this does not completely deter physicians. My most memorable moment in behavior therapy occurred when a patient was standing in line ahead of me in the grocery store. She picked out a pack of cigarettes, turned to me and said "I'm not in your office, I know what you're thinking and I'm not putting my smokes back." I smiled and said "not at all, I was going to suggest you take a whole carton, we just learned that patients who smoke have to see their physicians 50% more often for infections, and I could use the money."

She put the cigarettes back. It certainly isn't a technique that works on everyone, but I'm an in-your-face kind of physician. For Christmas that year she dropped off a card (citing 3 months without smoking) and two hand-made potholders.

People can change.

But why should you change to organic food? We established that for produce, there is no nutritional benefit to organic over conventional. Organic costs more and often spoils faster since it is a completely natural product.

The answer isn't because organic food has more nutrition. The answer is that organic food does not have toxins carried along with the nutrients.

The reason to eat organically is for what you are not getting – herbicides, pesticides, artificial fertilizers, genetic growth enhancers, cosmetic-enhancers, the list, as Dr Rachel Carson predicted more than half a century before, could be compiled in a "Who's Who" chemical compendium.

When you buy an apple, you should only be taking home an apple. You should only be eating an apple. You should only be absorbing an apple and your body should have nothing to deter it from absorbing all the nutrients it can from the apple. Any chemical that is *not* the apple is toxic to your body, and millenia of human genome ancestors have not evolved to make anything other than that apple safe and nutritious for you.

Our bodies are designed to handle eating some bugs, a bit of animal poop and fur, and some dust and dirt. It can handle most mold. There are plenty of bacteria that not only don't bother the body but actually enhance health and the immune system. The humans who encountered all those things and could not manage that amount of natural contamination died long before their reproductive years. In other words, humans weak to nature were not your ancestors. Embrace your ancestor's strengths. Those are *your* strengths.

What can't your body handle? It clearly cannot manage anything your ancestors did not encounter thousands of years ago. You can embrace the natural strength of your ancestors or your family can be the experiment for the future millennia of humans. My medical advice: trust the genome from your ancestors that made your existence possible. Avoid your body's weaknesses.

Not only Toxins are Toxic

"Don't eat anything your great-great grandmother wouldn't recognize as food. There are a great many food-like items in the supermarket your ancestors wouldn't recognize as food... stay away from these."
—Michael Pollan

Mr. Pollan gives excellent advice in the quote, and it is an excellent and safe starting point for diet detoxification. As before, until we define what we are talking about, we are not communicating well. So what is a toxin?

A toxin has the primary effect of interfering with body function in a harmful or deadly manner. The primary purpose of a toxin is to hurt or kill a living thing (that could be an insect, a weed, a rat or you). The most highly effective toxins are called poisons. Cyanide is a toxin and an effective poison.

Some toxins can be used in very small amounts for overall beneficial effects even though their primary purpose is death. For example, Coumadin is a prescription blood thinner also used as rat poison. In very tiny doses, Coumadin thins the blood by interfering with specific protein metabolism in the liver, treating or preventing otherwise life-threatening blood clots. By stopping one mechanism in the body, the patient is spared the natural course of death from a clotting cascade. It is an excellent medication for this as it is inexpensive, can be monitored for both effect and safety, and if overdosed has readily available antidotes.

Tox**ic**, as opposed to tox**in**, is the dose or amount of any substance that disrupts normal biochemical function in a manner that is more harmful than helpful.

Caffeine, for example, is not a toxin but can be toxic. In small amounts it can improve certain body functions by inhibiting the breakdown of a particular energy pathway (cyclic AMP). In larger amounts that same effect causes extreme overstimulation of the nervous system causing anxiety and tremors (this would be a toxic effect) and at higher levels death by disruption of heart rhythm.

All drugs, vitamins and supplements are toxic when the concentration in the body is high enough. If there was no toxicity and only upside, you wouldn't need doctors or pharmacists, and we could start training barbers to resume their past history as surgeons. Health providers learn to manage, sometimes with exhaustive calculations, the toxicity of medicinal substances by applying a concept (which is now measureable) called "therapeutic window."

The therapeutic window ranges from the lowest amount of substance needed to have a desired effect to the highest amount that can be given without increasing risk of death. (This isn't a Pharmacology textbook, so simply accept the concept for this book's purpose.) Ninety-nine percent of a pharmacist's job is making sure patients stay within this safety net — which is why they are deservedly well-paid and why I am always pleased when a pharmacist calls me for clarification. You need this safety net. Never use a "cheap" internet source for your medication.

Here is where I lose people: EVERYTHING has a therapeutic index.

Not enough oxygen – you die. Too much oxygen – you die.

Not enough sunshine – you die (without another vitamin D source). Too much sunshine – you die.

Not enough water – you die. Too much water – you die.

Not enough Tylenol – you have a headache for a few more hours. Two Tylenol – your headache goes away faster. One bottle of Tylenol – you die.

Not enough Glyphosate, MCPA, Pendimethlin, Malathion, Trichlorfon — your food costs more. Too much Glyphosate, MCPA, Pendimethlin, Malathion, Trichlorfon — you die. You can insert any insecticide/herbicide/fungicide in this paragraph, I had no intent of exonerating unmentioned manufacturers.

The difference between natural substances and created (artificial) substances is that you MUST have some of the natural substances to survive. Of the natural substances you need to survive, only humans who tolerated a wide range of exposure survived to reproduce, and their legacy to us is the strength in our genes to safely use a broad range of naturally-occurring substances.

Recall our discussion of enzymes. When any substance introduced to the body is either man-made or at a concentration higher than occurs in nature (such as a vitamin pill) there are 30, 000 factorial combination of ways to hurt that cell. That's 30,000! for the math geeks in the audience, and infinity for the non-math geeks. For practical purposes, just think of 30.000! as the biggest number you can conceptualize. The point? The ways you can harm your body's function is so large that there is no way to know how a manmade or supraphysiologic (higher than found normally in the body) dose of natural compound will affect you. But you can be certain of this: Not all the ways it affects you are healthful. Pesticides are not only man-made, but designed specifically to interfere with certain enzymes.

By now one might think "Dr Frank is anti-pesticide." You would be incorrect. I am anti-chemical if that chemical has a great likelihood of harming people. It is not quite as easy as all pesticides are always bad all the time.

Recall DDT. We decried the DDT pesticide prematurely (which was comparatively safer than some current insecticides) when it could have spared millions of people from malaria death and arguably more from starvation. Clearly there are occasions when chemical intervention in our environment makes sense. If I have to choose between saving friable wild bird eggs and human children in continental Africa, I'll pick saving the human children in Africa every time. We also received large exceptional brains from our ancestors and we should use them. Few things are always good or always bad.

In Northern America, where the issue is self-inflicted diseases and an excess of food, using artificial chemical manipulation is unnecessary and has not been proven safe. We don't need more food or less expensive food. We are not starving nor is anyone starving in the United States. Political activists lie to you — one should never equate "hungry" with "starving." It is medically desirable to be hungry; it is not desirable to be starving. Increasingly, research indicates we are eating far too much food far too often — being hungry and *not* satisfying that hunger strengthens the body and may also be key to healthier aging[11], stopping cancer and slowing heart disease.[12,13,14]

---

[11] Brandhorst S. Choi IY, Wei M. et al. Cell Metabolism 2015 22(1):86-99.

[12] Longo V, Mattson M. Cell Metabolism. 2014 19(2):181-192.

[13] Harvie M, Pegington M, Mattson M. et al. Int J Obesity. 2011;35(5):714-727.

That said, Northern America is suffering from malnutrition not hunger. This malnutrition is not due to insufficient quantity of food — but quite the opposite. It is due to nutritional imbalance not optimized for body biochemistry. More on this in another chapter.

Thus we have *toxins*, the primary purpose of which is to kill, and *toxic*, the effect anything can have when present in too high an amount for a living organism.

Some toxic levels are common sense and experiential. Too long in the sun – your skin gets sore or hot and you know to avoid it. Too much alcohol and your thoughts get fuzzy and you know to stop or you'll get sick. Our genetic legacy allows us to experience nature in moderation and stay healthy through our reproductive years despite some minor misadventures.

Our senses allow us, like all animals, to learn: avoiding stimuli (experiences) giving us a negative reaction and returning to stimuli giving us pleasure. The stimulus must be linked in the animals' brain to the stimulus event, which means a short time between stimulus and effect. Unlike other animals, however, humans can discern two or more outcomes. A stimulus can generate a mixture of positive and negative effects. Humans can further imagine an immediate event causing a future positive or

---

[14] Cheng X, Cai Y. Fan P, et al. Diabetes. 2015 64(5):1576-1590.

negative effect. It is this trait that allows concern over a positive effect (the pleasure of eating inexpensive tasty food) and a future negative effect (the chemicals in or on the food causing poor health).

Artificial exposures (or very rarely occurring natural exposures) are not experiential or common sense. Unless it impacts our senses in a toxic way, the experience outcome is unknown. This is important — our bodies cannot know how a small substance affects our body over time unless there is an immediate feedback. Therefore we cannot "learn" to avoid something from an experience that provides no feedback to us. This book is your feedback.

Small amounts of toxins over time can produce a toxic effect. If the body does not know it is experiencing a negative effect, it cannot act to diminish the exposure. When it comes to all things unknown, it is unwise to assume that an unknown is safe. If you are buying it from a seller you cannot easily sue for harm (which encompasses internet purchases in most cases), it is not safe.

Too much of a bad thing is worse

"If you can't pronounce it, don't eat it."
—Common sense

"Eat of the good things which We have provided for you."
—Quran 2:172

Read the label. Your last defense against artificial substances is the law that mandates everything knowingly added to an edible product must list the ingredients on the label. According to researchers at the University of Alabama, the average American consumes fourteen pounds of artificial chemicals each year. Your ancestors consumed no artificial chemicals ever. READ THE LABEL.

If, after reading this book, you still decide to eat processed food and food-like products, then at least read the label. For most people, if you cannot pronounce it, don't eat it. For those of you who have had college-level chemistry courses and can pronounce it, you are not using the intelligence your ancestors provided and I'll make a lot of money seeing you in my clinic for your preventable chronic medical conditions so give this book to someone who will use it.

Everything ingested must be broken down into some basic components for your body to use in growth, repair and sustenance. When the body ingests naturally occurring fats, protein and carbohydrates in commonly occurring quantities and mixtures, all the metabolic pathways can function appropriately. When faced with a substance which it cannot break down (or a substance in quantities far exceeded natural concentrations), the body has only three options: do not absorb it; absorb and attempt to eliminate it; absorb it and store it somewhere.

Most persons are aware of the body's "do not absorb" reactions: vomiting and diarrhea. This often occurs when the body finds concentrations far in excess of what exists commonly in nature. Most cases of "stomach flu" or "24 hour flu" are not from the flu or any other virus. It is the body's elimination of toxic levels of biologic waste (food poisoning) or rancid oils. Most short-lived episodes of diarrhea have similar causes — bad food. Your body is quite good at eliminating bad food.

We use the "do not absorb" reaction to our benefit as well. If you eat something that cannot be absorbed by the body but does absorb water (wood dust – the most common ingredient in over the counter constipation remedies), it moves through your intestines absorbing water and pushing everything along nicely until you have a good-sized stool the next day. If you eat something that cannot be absorbed but does not absorb and hold water (soap – the most common over the counter laxative or "stool softener"), it gives you looser stools. If you eat something that pulls excess water into your gut so quickly it cannot be rebalanced (magnesium salts – a common laxative used to produce short term diarrhea), you have liquid stools.

Those substances are not desired by the body, so it refuses to absorb them. None of those substances promoting regular bowel movements are needed if your body is getting appropriate nourishment. Your body is trying to protect itself by refusing to absorb useless substances.

But what happens if your body *does* absorb a useless substance or a toxin?

Then your body must find another way to get rid of the useless substance.

Detoxification is a much more complicated process. The main pathways for detoxification are in the liver. Except for the brain, the liver is the most fascinating and complex organ in the body. Through the biochemistry of the liver, toxins and useless substances are modified so that the modified substance can be either excreted in the feces, urine, sweat or breath. If the liver can make it water soluble or gas soluble, it will. Once soluble, the simple acts of breathing, sweating, urinating or breastfeeding will eliminate the toxins. If it cannot be excreted, it is stored – primarily in fats. While there are some exceptions (heavy metals such as mercury and lead are examples), this describes the body detoxification method.

The liver, like all tissues, becomes less efficient with age and insult. The biochemistry of the liver relies on numerous cofactors. The detoxification pathways are standardized — there is not a special enzymatic pathway for each toxin. This means the more toxins you give the liver, the greater the backload of toxin that builds up. There is even some protection against this. The liver can be *induced* or encouraged to make more of the needed detoxifying enzymes by some toxins. Some of these inducers are pharmaceutical medications and supplements. But other pharmaceuticals can down-regulate or *reduce* the detoxification pathways.

To complicate matters, while the liver has some control over the enzymes, many enzymes require co-factors — often in the form of micronutrients such as vitamins and mineral elements. Further complicating the matter is that over-abundance of some co-factors can interfere with other enzymes and other co-factors. More on this toxic effect of too many vitamins in another chapter.

Rather than despair, simply recall the liver will do just fine if not given more toxins than our ancestors gave to their livers.

Potentially overwhelming toxins to the liver include: pharmaceutical medications, over-the-counter medications, smoking, charbroiled food, pesticides, herbicides, fungicides, some plastics, Styrofoam, synthetic hormones, orally administered hormones, food dyes, artificial sweeteners, preservatives, and most every food supplement or vitamin taken above physiologic amounts (essentially all supplements).

Helpful to the liver (in clearing toxins that have been modified) are the cruciferous vegetables. Your mother was right: eat your broccoli and brussel sprouts.

This does not mean never ingesting a toxin. Your liver can handle most naturally-occurring toxins in physiologic amounts without incident.

This does mean more care should be taken in avoiding toxins that do not exist in nature. The most reasonable approach is to eliminate the toxins that cannot possibly benefit the body: food additives, Styrofoam, plastics, artificial sweeteners, food dyes and supplements. Also avoid anything ending in "cide" (which means death, incidentally). It definitely means taking more care in reducing exposure to nonphysiologic (toxic) levels of supplements.

Never assume a vitamin or mineral is low simply because you feel a particular way. There are myriad reasons for any particular symptom. Never assume an herbal supplement will solve a problem. It can mask symptoms, worsen conditions, interfere with prescription medications, and with some herbs cause cancer, blood clotting disorders and liver disease. While many pharmaceutical medications are patterned after or are chemical analogues of naturally occurring compounds, remember that taking a supplement is not necessarily safer than taking a pharmaceutical pill. Unlike a supplement, we know exactly what is in a pharmaceutical pill. Once the list of artificial toxins and non-physiologic toxic compounds are eliminated from your diet, you may not need all of your pharmaceuticals. That important decision should be discussed with your doctor at that time.

What your doctor likely cannot help you with is detoxifying. That is simply a weakness of medical training or rather, a weakness of people that is not addressed adequately in medical training to banish it from healthcare professionals thought processes.

The assumption that to be sold food must be safe is erroneous. There are no long-term studies proving that humans cannot be harmed by accumulated man-made compounds in our environment. Compared to pharmaceutical regulations, the safety requirements for food, food additives, pesticides, drugs given to farm animals and food containers are laughable. The answer is not to increase the regulations, but rather to increase consumer knowledge.

We can measure a substance in humans that only exists in, for example, plastic coated cans and plastic bottles, such as Bisphenol – A (BPA). We know that BPA encourages fat production; humans can either eliminate that from their food choice or continue to accumulate the fat associated with BPA and the hormone imbalance that extra fat and BPA generates.

We can determine that man-made pesticides and herbicides (all of them) have hormonal (usually estrogen-like) effects in humans and blocks normal thyroid function, and we know that estrogen-like effects and thyroid disruption can increase some cancers, modify behavior, increase obesity and decrease sperm count. Humans can either eliminate that from their food choice by buying organic produce or continue to experience the effects.

We can determine that food additives cause cancer. The known cancer-causing nitrites[15] are listed directly on bacon and sausage packages. Some people choose to eat them anyway. We also know that eating fresh produce can reduce cancer risk[16,17,18]. Some people choose to avoid fresh produce[19].

We can determine that inhaling burned leaves (or anything burned) produces carcinogens that when inhaled cause cancer, weaken immune systems, harm developing babies and weaken skin structure. It is listed directly on the package. Some people choose to smoke anyway.

Some of the harmful effects of man-made chemicals are listed and available via Occupational Safety and Health Administration (OSHA). You paid for this information with your taxes and yet likely never used it. People, sometimes the people actually spraying the produce and weeds, are not aware of the dangers despite walking by posted chemical safety sheets every day. Sometimes they become aware in the Emergency Room with an acute

[15] Inoue-Choi M, Jones RR, Anderson KE, et al. Nitrate and nitrite ingestion and risk of ovarian cancer among postmenopausal women in Iowa. Int J Cancer. 2015 Jul 1;137(1):173-82. doi: 10.1002/ijc.29365. Epub 2014 Dec 8.
[16] Pavia M, Pileggi C, Nobile CG, Angelillo IF. Association between fruit and vegetable consumption and oral cancer: a meta-analysis of observational studies. Am J Clin Nutr. 2006 May;83(5):1126-34
[17] Lunet N, Lacerda-Vieira A, Barros H. Fruit and vegetables consumption and gastric cancer: a systematic review and meta-analysis of cohort studies. Nutr Cancer. 2005;53(1):1-10. MMWR. July 10, 2015 / 64(26);709-713
[18] Gandini S, Merzenich H, Robertson C, Boyle P. Meta-analysis of studies on breast cancer risk and diet: the role of fruit and vegetable consumption and the intake of associated micronutrients. Eur J Cancer. 2000 Mar;36(5):636-46.
[19] Moore LV. Adults Meeting Fruit and Vegetable Intake Recommendations — United States, 2013.

overexposure, other times in the cancer center from chronic exposure.

People already have a choice. The reactive cycle that needs breaking is a concept of treating the symptom of one condition with another chemical that itself causes toxicity. While people like to blame physicians for this (and we are part of the problem), it is a rare patient that walks in to my office who is NOT already taking twice as many supplements as prescriptions, willfully loading their body with manmade toxins daily beginning with their very first cup of non-organic coffee and artificial creamer with artificial sweetener wanting to know why they are sick, tired and fat before they head to McDonald's for lunch.

Common sense and caring for yourself doesn't come in a pill. Where doctors deserve blame is in failing to educate themselves and then their patients by pointing out, as painful as it is, that unhealthy choices are the problem and that our out-the-door advice such as "stop smoking, eat less and exercise" is ineffective[20].

But that is what we are taught. We give them a pill to lower their cholesterol, a shot to lower their blood sugar, a diet pill so they will skip their only salad at noon, a

---

[20] Dombroski SU, Knittle K, Avenall A, Araujo-Soares V, Sniehotta FF. Long-term maintenance of weight loss with non-surgical interventions in obese adults: systematic review and meta-analysis of randomized controlled trials. BMJ 2014;348:g2646.

thyroid pill at a tiny dose so the patient can blame their weight on their thyroid, a blood pressure pill because their heart has to pump too hard to get blood through all the fat, a water pill because their ankles swell due to eating salt-laden snacks and canned foods, a pain pill because their back hurts from carrying around an extra person or two for decades, a depression pill because they don't like the life they've chosen, and a sleeping pill because their ribcage can no longer hold back the fat when they sleep so they need a CPAP machine to prevent sleep apnea but without a sleeping pill they cannot tolerate the machine's facemask.

That sadly describes the majority of patients I have seen in California, Illinois, Montana and Michigan[21]. I am displeased with that because I want people to have a normal life, and what I described, although common, is neither normal nor due to patients simply eating too much and not getting sufficient exercise. The obesity epidemic in America today, the unhealthiness of America today is in part due to the toxins we choose to ingest every day.

Your body doesn't care if it has to detoxify a supplement, prescription, pesticide or cigarette. It is ALL a disruption in body chemistry. If supplements were safe, there

---

[21] Although work in Kansas was primarily research-based; there is no reason to suspect patients in KS are any different however.

wouldn't be data showing that persons who take supplements die sooner than persons who do not take supplements[22]. And there are many such studies.

Helping your liver detoxify your body is also a choice.

Recall that the liver prefers to detoxify by making compounds water soluble. Once water soluble, you simply need to urinate or sweat it out. Drink more water — without any additives and out of a container that is BPA-free. Don't get dehydrated. Start yoga and walk daily. If you have access to a dry sauna, use it at least three times a week until beads of sweat form on your skin — then shower off quickly. You'll continue to sweat more, and your clothes will absorb those toxins. Don't wear those clothes again until after you've washed them.

When the liver cannot make a compound water soluble, it stores it in fat. You need to get rid of the stored fat gradually. If you lose it quickly, you will feel horrible as you are releasing toxins back into your circulation. Given to the liver slowly, some of these toxins can be excreted via the bile system and bound into the fiber in the feces.

There must be a lot of fiber in the feces to absorb these toxins. Assuming you have no medical contraindications, the best way to accomplish this is to eat an organic

---

[22] Dachner N, Mendelson R, Sacco J, Tarasuk V. An examination of the nutrient content and on-package marketing of novel beverages. *App Physiol Nut Metab.* 2015 January . www.ncbi.nlm.nih.gov/pubmed/25577949.

vegetarian diet supplemented with some organic flaxseed mixed ground to unground about 4:1. This dietary period should last at least four weeks. Know that the diet associated with the longest and healthiest life in humans is vegetarian. In the event that this is not an option, then the only animal products consumed can be organic cultured dairy. Cultured is dairy that has been fermented by bacteria; a common example is yoghurt. For additional information on cultured foods, read the chapter on fermentation.

There must be beneficial gut microorganisms to ensure detoxification of gut toxins. If you have been on antibiotics within the past six months, restoring normal gut microbes is important. Incorporate naturally fermented products with active cultures into the diet. Examples are yoghurt, kefir, miso, organic unfiltered apple cider, sauerkraut and kimchee. Most rural persons may have to make sauerkraut and kimchee themselves. Larger cities will offer these options in their grocery area, most often in the refrigerated produce section. Regardless of whether you purchase your produce or ferment it yourself, ensure that is *not* pasteurized or otherwise heat-processed after the helpful bacteria have grown. Additionally, persons adhering to a vegan diet long-term need to educate themselves regarding protein sufficiency in vegan diets. You don't need animal products to get sufficient protein, but you should understand how the plant products can be combined to ensure your body receives sufficient protein components.

"Then God said, 'Behold, I have given you every plant yielding seed that is on the surface of all the earth, and every tree which has fruit yielding seed; it shall be food for you; and to every beast of the earth and to every bird of the sky and to everything that moves on the earth which has life, I have given every green plant for food;' and it was so." — Genesis 1:29-30. The Bible.

Supplement companies count on your ignorance

"Stupid is as stupid does."
—Forrest Gump

"Tell me what you think about this: if we needed vitamin
pills to live we'd all be dead."
—Otto J. Hetzner

My grandfather had an interesting and usually kind way of
expressing his opinion. In this instance, telling me in
medical school that vitamin pills aren't necessary or
humans wouldn't have lived long enough for us to be
around to discuss it. I should have listened to him.
The persistent myth that supplements, whether vitamins
or herbal or combinations thereof, will improve health
and well-being is understandable but false. What are
supplements? In the United States, dietary supplements
are considered food; supplements are intended to provide
nutrients that may otherwise not be consumed in
sufficient quantities. As food, no medical claims can be
made. Vitamins, minerals and herbs are all supplements.
Some supplements are marketed as vitamins while others
are marketed for health-related reasons. The marketing is
always false from the standpoint of science: no
supplement has ever been shown to improve health

unless there has been a laboratory-confirmed deficiency *or* we are using the supplement for its toxic effect.

All supplements, like all pharmaceuticals, can cause side effects and generally increase the toxic burden on your body. There are no studies showing that supplements improve health, but there are many studies proving that supplements increase risk of death[23,24,25]. That is worth repeating: taking supplements increases your risk of death and disease. Trying to prevent cancer with vitamin and mineral supplements will increase[26], not decrease your cancer risk[27].

That is simply science. Denying facts does not make the facts go away. It merely proclaims the denier's stupidity. One can deny the speed of light, the force of gravity or the safety and effectiveness of vaccines, but that does not change the facts or lessen the impact of the facts upon one's life.

[23] Wien TW, Pike E, Wisloff T, Staff A et al. Cancer risk with folic acid supplements: a systematic review and meta-analysis. BMJ Open. 2012;2:e000653.

[24] Druesne-Pecollo N, Latino-Martel P, Norat T, et al. Beta-carotene supplementation and cancer risk: a systematic review and meta-analysis of randomized controlled trials. Int J Cancer. 2010;127:172-184.

[25] Vinceti M, Dennert G, Crespi CM, et al. Selenium for preventing cancer. Cochrane Database Syst Rev. 2014;3:CD005195.

[26] Perera RM, Bardeesy N. Cancer: When antioxidants are bad. Nature 2011, 43-44. 475. doi:10.1038/475043a

[27] Klein EA, Thompson IM Jr, Tangen CM, et al. Vitamin E and the risk of prostate cancer: the Selenium and Vitamin E Cancer Prevention Trial (SELECT). JAMA. 2011:306:1549-1556.

Supplements are dangerous primarily because people think of them as safe. They are not. People think supplements are safe because medical science can isolate a substance and show that persons consuming the substance *as part of the food from which it naturally occurs* have less of a particular disease or condition. Alternatively, medical science can show that a *deficiency* of a particular substance can cause a disease or medical condition.

The error is to think that by *over*-replacing a substance we are helping the body or by replacing a substance *by itself* we are helping the body.

Academics called this reductionist thinking (or in this case, reductionist nutrition), and it is flawed. Normal people call this stupid because it is flawed.

Supplement manufacturers call this windfall profits. Because this type of flawed thinking is closely tied to emotion, it allows for easy marketing to both academics and normal people. Emotion can trump logic. Let's explore why supplements are such an easy way for companies to profit from human weakness.

We are encouraged to believe that pills sold legally in the United States are safe when we actually are in a *buyer beware* market. There is no legal requirement that any food source, which includes all vitamins and herbal supplements, have safety parameters. There are no requirements for standardization. There are no requirements for effectiveness. There are no requirements for consistency between pills, let alone bottles. There are no requirements at all save that which protects you from buying anything else at the store.

The beauty of supplements is this: as long as they make no direct health claims, the manufacturers do not need to follow any medication laws. If ever there was a case for the effectiveness of marketing and advertising, health and beauty supplements win with no close second.

Medical and regulatory people understand this. For example, to a physician there is a huge difference between a cream that says "reduces wrinkles and age spots by 38%" and a cream that says "reduces the *appearance* of wrinkles and fine lines within 10 days". The first claim is measurable and objective – it is *real*. The second statement isn't a claim in the legal sense at all. It is an opinion that is not measurable and is purely subjective. The FDA can remove the first product from the market if the product does not meet the claim. The FDA can remove the first product from the market if, despite the claim, users have a higher risk of skin cancer. A consumer can bring a successful legal suit against a company if a FDA approved product does not meet claims. The FDA and the consumer have no power against the second company any more than it would if you bought an orange and smeared it on your wrinkles and got no change in your skin appearance from your perspective.

Medical products that have an impact on specific and measurable health parameters have clinical data proving those parameters filed and reviewed by the FDA. After such review, the U.S. government allows specific proven medical claims to be advertised about the products. Supplements do not. Supplements have no government or agency review. Nothing.

Supplement manufacturers also know the power of suggestion. So do physicians. We call this the placebo effect and when it comes to feelings (reduced pain, better sleep, improved libido, less congestion) we know the power of the mind can effect a 5 – 10% change in a positive way *even if* the drug given to the patient is a blank (placebo) — as long as patients *expect* it to have that effect.

If you tell two groups of patients they are taking a sleeping pill but you actually give one of the groups a sugar pill at bedtime, the group that took the sugar pill will report up to 10% better sleep simply because they *expected* the pill to help them sleep. The more you trust the influencer, the better the placebo effect. If your best friend or favorite nurse asks you to try a sleeping pill and gives you a sugar pill, it will work better than if your ex-wife's lawyer tells you the same thing.

The placebo effect is not limited to inactive or weak substances. Pharmaceutical medications get the benefit (or detriment) from the power of suggestion as well.

So if supplements can make no real health claims and many simply rely on placebo effect and marketing, is there any harm?

Yes. Supplement harm extends beyond the proven risk of cancer; supplements interact with other essential nutrients in unintended ways that can render some micronutrients less effective and can be harmful to the body systems in far too many ways to track[28,29].

An average American spends about $400 a year on supplements with no health claims yet expecting health benefits. They are, from one point of view, being swindled out of money that could be used to actually help them in other ways. In many cases, the money spent does not even purchase the intended supplement at all, as was recently demonstrated by the FDA when several large chain drug stores were inspected for food labeling.

---

[28] Nutrition and the Immune System: A Review of Nutrient-Nutrient Interactions. Kubena KS; McMurray DN. Journal of the American Dietetic Association 96. 1996: 1156-64.
[29] Role of Nutrition in the Drug Metabolizing System. Campbell TC; Hayes JR. Pharmacological Reviews.26. 1974:171-97.

What they found were herbal supplements that did not contain the labeled herbs on the ingredient list but dried common house plants[30]. These were major brand stores that tout their supplements: Walgreens, Walmart, GNC and Target. Sometimes the herbal products in reality contain a mixture of pharmaceutical drugs.[31] Imagine you believe you are taking something to help your health and you actually ingest a medication to which you are allergic. Or worse.

If this happened at a restaurant, most people would be livid enough to never eat there again. Imagine getting ground housecat instead of ground beef. But no such rational behavior occurs with supplements. Consumers still want to believe in magic even when it turns out to be dried bougainvillea.

Lack of effectiveness aside, while supplements cannot make health claims, they also cannot make safety claims. As a physician, this is my greatest concern.

All substances in excess of levels the body can immediately use are toxic. Extra or unnecessary substances must be eliminated or, in the case of energy and a few fat-soluble substances, stored as fat.

---

[30] http://inhabitat.com/fda-finds-herbal-supplements-at-four-major-retailers-contain-asparagus-houseplants-and-no-herbs/
[31] http://www.fda.gov/Safety/Recalls/ucm469981.htm

When the body machinery is functioning at peak for any particular biochemical process, giving it more starting material or more ancillary materials will not make the biochemical process better. Think of a biochemical process as the running motor of a car. Adding gas to the car that is already running will not make the engine run better. Adding oil to the car that is already running will not make it run better. Conversely, if we add too much gas to the running car, the tank spills over and we damage the car's paint. Run even more over and some of the car's tire gets dissolved by the gas. Run too much over and risk an explosion that can destroy the car. The car needs even less oil. Add too much oil while running the car and you can start a fire or even destroy the engine. Guessing what supplements to add to the oil could make the oil *less* effective and ultimately destroy the motor early.

A similar concept applies to your body. Take for example the effect of excesses on your external body, excesses you can actually see. If you bleach or perm your hair, why not leave the chemical on twice as long? Won't the result be twice as good? Why not wash your hair ten times more and dry it with 100 times the heat? Why stop with an exfoliating sponge when sandpaper can take off more layers of dead skin more completely? Wouldn't you look more beautiful if you covered your face with the entire make-up bottle? Why stop with two spritzes of cologne when you have an entire bottle?

When it involves the body, more is rarely better. When body has enough of something, more is *never* better. The biochemistry of our body was optimized for normal naturally occurring concentrations of everything it needs. Guessing at supplements will *never* help the body and usually harm the body.

When a healthcare provider feels you may be deficient in a substance, we can test the levels. If you are deficient, we can replace it. In some medical instances, there is short-term benefit in over-replacing to ensure we avoid permanent harm. Pregnancy and alcoholism are the two common examples where we over-replace for a year (pregnancy) to reduce, for example, the risk of birth defects or replace for a few weeks (alcoholism) to reduce the risk of brain damage. We over-replace some patients short term to prevent death or disability that could otherwise occur as a long-term outcome.

Another example is vitamin D. In some instances, such as kidney failure common in diabetics, we measure and replace one or more forms of vitamin D. In patients with little sun exposure, we measure and replace vitamin D if needed. In patients who have had their stomach removed to cure their obesity, we measure and replace several types of nutrients. We measure to minimize harm to the patient because even vitamins are toxins when taken at doses above those needed for the body to function. More isn't better. In some cases, more can actually kill you. Iron and Vitamin A are great examples of highly toxic nutrients — those which have a smaller therapeutic window.

As bad as vitamin supplements can be, herbal supplements are much worse because herbal supplements have less standardization and can interact badly with prescription medication and other food supplements.

That does not mean herbal supplements cannot be used. It is important to understand that supplements are simply unregulated medications. My non-pregnant adult patients have that option within the following safety parameters:

1. The herbal supplement must contain only one ingredient.
2. The ingredient must be standardized in an acceptable manner.
3. The herbal supplement must be manufactured (not just distributed) in the United States or Canada.
4. The dose cannot be changed without consulting with me.
5. Whenever possible, organically grown supplements processed to pharmaceutical grade standards are purchased.

This assures me some level of safety, for supplements can be as toxic as prescription medications. The rules above impose upon supplements the same reduction of toxicity that is already applied to prescription medication. I draw the supplement efficacy data from biochemical equivalence in structure and whenever possible, clinical trials. There are a few well-designed clinical studies that have been done on herbal supplements.

In brief these have shown that St. John's wort can be used in mild to moderate depression, red yeast rice can be used in some forms of high cholesterol and green tea can reduce mild anxiety. The effect is not as strong as the pharmaceuticals (which were patterned after the active ingredients in the herbs then modified to make it patentable) but then neither are the side-effects. Other herbs have demonstrated danger without benefit. Some of these are gingko biloba, country mallow, usnea, chaparral, bitter orange and ephedra. Other supplements such as cinnamon, chromium and Coenzyme Q 10 have shown some benefit but only in specific medical conditions or in combination with certain pharmaceutical treatments.

Unfortunately, medical training in the United States does not teach this and I have primarily my European and Asian colleagues (and several herbal texts they and my wiccan patients threw my way) to thank for broadening my experience. It is an unwise patient that forces a doctor into an area the doctor does not understand or have experience with. Respect your physician's limitations. Some basics:

- ✓ You do NOT have to use herbal supplements to achieve state of the art medical care.
- ✓ You DO increase your risks when you bring unknowns into your treatment regimen. When any doctor incorporates herbal supplements, particularly if you are on other medications, drug interactions occur.
- ✓ Do not guess and do not self-medicate. If you have a condition that is associated with a specific deficiency, your physician can use clinical evidence and guidelines to minimize harm. In many instances, the specific level of vitamin or mineral can be measured and adjusted in a personalized way.
- ✓ Do not use the Internet to self-diagnose. In 30 years I have only had one patient self-diagnose correctly via the Internet. But then she also paid money for laboratory testing - over $300 more than it would have cost if I had ordered the laboratory testing.
- ✓ There have never been health break-throughs despite media hype. True medical advances occur

in very small steps, whether it be a pharmaceutical or a food supplement.

I have had patients with allergic reactions to Internet supplements advertised and sold on the sites they visited. I have had patients forego proven medical therapies for life-threatening conditions, falsely believing that supplements can heal without side-effects despite scientific evidence to the contrary. I had a patient in Chicago die from metastatic breast cancer that we could have stopped, but she persisted with her supplements until the cancer spread widely. I had two patients in California nearly die from contaminants in a common marine lipid supplement designed to lower cholesterol.

Supplements can be just as dangerous as prescription drugs, more so when patients miss the opportunity of a proven drug therapy that, all things being equal, could have improved or saved their lives.

For those persons who feel supplements are a critical part of their daily food intake despite facts, a logical extension of that argument is that all supplements should be chewed and tasted in original form, not swallowed in a pill to bypass ancestral defenses. Supplements that cannot be chewed and swallowed without an adverse taste reaction (without covering up the taste with dilution or sweetening) would not have been consumed by our ancestors. If it wouldn't have been eaten by our ancestors, it has toxicity in our body.

An important side note for persons who have been duped into thinking that they must take supplements daily: if you have been taking high doses of certain supplements for a long time, it can be dangerous and even fatal to abruptly stop. In much the same way that abruptly stopping chronic alcohol abuse (a supplement) can cause seizures and death and stopping certain herbals can cause seizures and death, it would be unwise to simply stop supplements without physician guidance. Abrupt withdrawal of certain chronic toxic compounds can be harmful. Gradual reduction over several weeks is likely a safer route unless a very deadly substance is taken. I encourage readers to consult with a physician or naturopath regarding this weaning process.

When my patients stop smoking, a common complaint is that they catch colds more often. What really happens is that they cough more because they no longer have toxic smoke killing off the lining of their airways. The purpose of that lining is to eject toxins from the lungs. So they cough up the grey (sometimes black) toxin-laden sputum. They aren't getting sick, but they sometimes feel crappy while in the process of eliminating those toxins.

When patients stop high doses of kava, they can have seizures. Stopping high doses of minerals can precipitate muscle cramps. High doses of caffeine or ephedra abruptly stopped will cause headaches. The list is extensive and the point is simply that in reducing supplements you should consult a physician or a licensed naturopath.

For some, adopting a life free of supplements is emotionally stressful. Having been a student of Dr. Linus Pauling's teachings[32] —the brilliant biochemist — I found it difficult to eject supplements from my life despite seeing data that his reductionist views of nutrition were flawed. I had followed his advice for years personally, and while intellectually I knew the supplements should be stopped, I felt a strong emotional loss. Thus I made a schedule to continually decrease my supplements each month in both number and strength while monitoring my health. While self-disclosure is often frowned upon in medicine, you need to know that even the most highly educated persons struggle with this emotional addiction. Knowing is one thing, doing is another. (Remember what I said about the strength of marketing? It anchors on your emotions and traps you with emotion.)

Taste serves a protective mechanism by encouraging ingestion of substances pleasurable and discouraging substances triggering nociceptors (noci = harmful). The substances desired and tolerated by the body also change

[32] How to Live Longer and Feel Better. Pauling L. Avon Books. 1987.

during times of growth or pregnancy, driving the desire for substances of higher need. Foods that taste sweet in nature are never poisonous; foods that taste bitter can be poisonous.

Most parents can attest to this. It is easier to get a child to eat raw fruit than raw salad greens. Chemical heat or physical heat triggers nociceptors —children have to be taught to like hot foods — whether by blowing frequently on hot food or taking tiny amounts of plants, like cayenne or jalapenos until their brains learn to tolerate these. Salt is a desirable taste until one takes too much or in too large a concentration, which triggers thirst to avoid fatal dehydration. Ancestors did not drink saltwater but may have used it to wash or flavor food.

Bitter and rancid tastes, which predominate when chewing unadulterated supplements, elicit a non-absorption response: spit it out or vomit later. A response to bitter can be overridden but rancid or putrid will result in a non-absorption response. This is not a conscious decision. Ancestors without these protective neural pathways died.

Fast food and processed food manufacturers understand this. The most addictive foods trigger more than one pleasure center. The most addictive foods use a combination of saturated fat, salt and sugar.

What other forms of supplementation imbalance the body?

Consider not only supplements purposefully taken by an individual but also the supplements added by others to the diet in our food and drink. For example, most grain products have vitamins added to either provide a marketing illusion of "better" or to improve a product's taste, look or feel. Common examples are folic acid, bromine and fluoride.

Those who know about the genetic manipulation of wheat and eat it anyway may not care about the additives. Folic acid (Folate), a vitamin critical to several enzymes in the body, is added to flour to reduce the risk of folate deficiency that can cause certain birth defects called neural tube defects. Well-intended as this may be, we have studies now that show folic acid supplementation increases the risk of some cancers. For women planning imminent pregnancy as for persons taking certain immunosuppressive medications, the benefit of supplements outweigh the risk. Otherwise, it is toxic — too much will disrupt body biochemistry.

Bromine is added to flour to improve the look and feel of baked goods. While linked with cancer in animal models, a bigger concern derives from the atomic table and analytical chemistry. It is likely to interfere with similarly charged trace elements that have a similar three-dimensional electron cloud (atomic) structure.

What essential elements can bromine mimic in this way? Chloride, which is so abundant in any diet that it bears no further discussion, and iodine, which is a rare element critical to thyroid-driven metabolism and a cofactor in at least one enzyme that helps prevent cancer. It is not unreasonable to link these various facts. Animals given bromine get more cancer. Bromine competes with iodine, and iodine then cannot fuel a cancer-inhibiting enzyme.

What else is even more ubiquitous in our diets since the 1940s and shares bromide and iodide characteristics? Fluoride. Here we have the well-intentioned public health push to prevent tooth decay. Laudable goal, short-term thinking. First public health added potassium iodide to all salt to prevent thyroid dysfunction, then it fluorinated public water supply to counter-act the iodine (unintentionally). Does fluoride reduce tooth decay? Most definitely. Does it interfere with other body biochemistry? Most definitely. Should adults be using fluoride? Most definitely not. Can you greatly reduce your fluoride intake even if you do not have well-water? Yes, but it will cost you.

If your adult teeth are prone to cavities, your dentist can address that. If fluoride is the prescribed treatment for you, then ask for it as drops you can control or as topical application in the form of prescription toothpaste or fluoride gel.

Fluoride should not be in our water. It should not be in everyone's toothpaste. It is a toxin (you read that correctly) that like any medication can be used in tiny doses when appropriate for medicinal purposes for a defined period of time and monitored by your dentist.

While some dentists will tow the American Dental Association (ADA) line, most that I have met are far more intelligent than the collective guidelines. Whenever any political health organization agrees with a government intervention that does not require the approval of the individual, be skeptical. I have served on enough well-meaning committees to know that a consensus opinion means there is disagreement by experts. If experts disagree, then data is usually insufficient to form a conclusive opinion. Consider a consensus opinion only a starting point, not the endgame. We are not done with either fluoride or consensus medical opinions. Read on.

Supplement Stupidity, part 2

"The doctor of the future will no longer treat the human frame with drugs, but rather will cure and prevent disease with nutrition." —Thomas Edison

People have been taught to think wrongly about food and the components that comprise their food. Food is not simply a collection of macro and micronutrients. Food is nutritious because of nature's complexity; our best science cannot replicate this complexity. But we can study it and the data from such studies is both amazing and concerning. Let's begin with a common apple.[33]

The science we call medicine utilizes the scientific method to eliminate or control all the variables concerning a medical question. With this tool, we have successfully found specific disease markers and can isolate specific infectious organisms. When there is one cause of a disease, such as a virus, bacteria, poison or antibodies against one's self, this tool works exceptionally well.

---

[33] Apples, Raw with skin. from Self magazine. nutritiondata.self.com/facts/fruits-and-fruit-juices/1809/2

However, method can fail us when a disease is multifactorial — caused by several things occurring at the same time, caused by more than one thing, or by things in sequence.

Cancer is a common example of this failure: there are many factors making cancer more likely. With few exceptions we cannot say "this one thing alone is the cause of cancer." Although we often hear "sunlight causes cancer" or "tobacco causes cancer." What is actually meant is "sunlight increases the likelihood of developing cancer", " tobacco increases the likelihood of developing cancer" and so on.

When it comes to cancer, physicians are very good at making these disclaimers. We understand that no one thing yields a 100% chance of cancer. We understand taking excess cancer risks is unwise. Additionally, we also understand cancer is not an "either-or" phenomenon — despite hearing the media and our patients exclaim such irrational claims daily.

"My sister tanned her whole life and she never got skin cancer" may be an accurate statement, but the next statement of "so I won't either" is silly. The first statement doesn't mean her sister won't get skin cancer (or perhaps she had it but died from something else) nor does it bear much relevance to whether or not the speaker will get skin cancer. If you told that same patient they could jump out of an airplane without a parachute and live because you know someone who jumped out of a parachute and lived, they'd rightfully look at you as an idiot. Yet the analogy would escape them.

In short, simply because something fails to occur 100% of the time does not mean it will occur 0% of the time.

Why bother with this example? Because physicians are quite good at understanding the complexities of human conditions when we expect the conditions to be complex and multi-factorial. But when the topic is nutrition, physicians are taught the simplistic reductionist view (which I will explain shortly) and therefore rightfully should often be considered unschooled insofar as nutrition is concerned.

That problem is compounded when the patients follow a similar pattern of illogic, leading to the common adage of the blind leading the blind. There is even a psychiatric label for shared delusions — folie à deux. This is not to imply that physicians are psychotic, merely to inform that we recognize delusions can be shared.

Back to the apple. If you ask anyone (even a physician) what's in an apple and they have had any indoctrination in conventional nutritional training, they offer something along the lines of "fiber, sugar and vitamins." If you ask them if an apple has vitamin C, they will say "no, but oranges do." If you ask them how they could replace the apple in their diet, they would say "with a fiber supplement and a vitamin pill." They would be wrong[34].

What was found in an apple is the equivalent of about 1500 mg of vitamin C (the common name for the chemical ascorbic acid). But this 1500mg *only* occurred when eaten raw. What was measured was not the chemical vitamin C, but rather the *activity* vitamin C has in the body. For the non-vitamin readers, 1500mg is more vitamin C than one can buy in a vitamin supplement.

Why the data discrepancy? The discrepancy occurred because when decomposing an apple in a laboratory, only about five mg of vitamin C is detected. This is not enough to even bother listing on a nutritional label. What the lab cannot tell us is how the thousands of other chemicals in the apple and in the human body interact to exponentially increase the antioxidant activity of vitamin C to meet the body's needs. And then some.

Yes the lab can measure how much vitamin C is detected in the apple. The lab cannot tell us how to replicate the apple's vitamin C activity in the body. The lab cannot tell us what all the other substances are in the apple in a way to safely meet the body's nutritional needs. What this

---

[34] Eberhardt MV, Lee CY, Liu RH. Antioxidant Activity of Fresh Apples. Nature 405. #6789. June 2000. 903-4.

means is that no supplements you take can replace the needed nutrition of actual food.

This is important: Supplements are inferior to actual food.

Let me share with you a tragic example. I have several patients who have what we refer to as short-gut syndrome. They were all tragic victims of trauma (one was a medical complication) who live without most of their intestines. They have had all but about fifteen inches of their twenty feet of gut removed. One military vet also lost his pancreas, turning him into an instant brittle diabetic to make matters more complex. These patients are tough to have even survived and I am proud of their tenacity. I am not proud, however, that nutritional supplement medicine has sentenced them to a horrid existence.

These patients are almost entirely dependent upon intravenous nutritional support and have been for years. We call this total parenteral nutrition (TPN) which in all studies is always inferior to gut feeding (food by mouth). These patients are sickly with sallow, droopy skin, sparse hair, dull eyes and are prone to many infections. They are considered disabled or handicapped. This is despite getting every nutrient (what normal persons would call supplements) that man-kind knows of directly into their blood stream! Further, we test their blood regularly and adjust nutrients, both macronutrients and micronutrients, to avoid any deficiencies or excess.

If I could use only one example to prove there is no way to replace or supplement nutrition and be healthy, it would be these poor patients.

No matter the number of supplements you take, you cannot replace the nourishment natural food has in your body. Real food can no more be replaced by supplements than your body can be replaced by carbon, hydrogen, nitrogen and oxygen. These four elements are what we would find in the lab if we decomposed your body to dust. If we add water back to the four elements from your decomposed body, would that turn the dust back into you? No, of course not. Nor can a handful of pills — the dust of the apple — nourish your body like the apple.

How did we get off the nutritional track?

What remains untaught for over a decade is that natural food is far more nutritious to the body when taken whole than when we reduce it to the chemicals that compose it. This has been called reductionist thinking. Reductionist thinking is a misapplication of the scientific method due to faulty assumptions. It is worse than simple nutrition reductionalism however. It is reductionist thinking followed by an inappropriate generalization.

In epidemiology, medicine looks at whether data is reasonably applicable to people that were not well-represented in the study. We call this generalizablity. We say a study is generalizable to the general population only if the study design proved valid in that population.

Here's a simple way to look at this. You do a study on some flatworms. The study finds that if you cut the worm in half, both halves live and grow into whole flatworms. This is actually true in nature and you can reproduce this study in the lab. Armed with this laboratory data, you decide to cut your dog in half so you can have twice as much dog to love. To your dismay, both halves of the dog die.

The mistake was to generalize the flatworm study to a population that was not represented in the study — a dog. The study was correct and factual. The error was applying — generalizing— the study findings to a population that was *not* studied. The flatworm study is said to be non-generalizable to dogs or other populations not well-represented in the original study.

In humans, application of study findings can be nearly as obvious as the flatworm example, but can at other times be difficult to discern. Sometimes lack of generalizability is obvious — a breast cancer study involving only women is not generalizable to men with breast cancer. Sometimes it is less clear, such as heart attack diagnosis criteria in diabetic white men being generalized to diabetic hispanic men. Sometimes even physicians struggle to explain that a study showing survival benefit for lowering blood pressure in high-risk patients can still mean danger for lowering blood pressure in normal-risk patients.

Back to the apple.

Reductionist thinking: If we study the apple and all other food a healthy person eats and reduce it down to its chemical substances (such as vitamin C); we can then assume that this complete list of chemical substances are all the nutrients necessary for a healthy human body. It is true we can break food down into components. It is false that this tells us what the complete *necessary* components are, in what combination or in which concentration the nutrients should be combined. It is a false assumption that in the process of breaking food down no compound was lost and no chemical structure was modified in a biologically meaningful way. It is also false to assume the matrix in which the components are combined — an apple — is unimportant. Reductionist thinking often asks the *wrong* question. What they should have asked is: how much vitamin C activity does an apple have in the human body? That is a much more complex question to correctly answer — or we would readily have much more data already.

Generalization thinking: For each compound found in the lab, we can reintroduce this chemical back into the body with the same effect. Further, we can combine all the individual lab data from each type of food and provide a complete list of all chemical substances found in food. We can tell people exactly how much of each nutrient their body needs to be healthy. It is true we can compile a list of the components from the laboratory. We can also identify how a *deficiency* of that compound can cause poor health. The false assumption is that putting the components from the lab back into the body will produce good health. Further, it has been proven that supplementing —the opposite of deficiency— is actually harmful to health. Generalization fails when, like Reductionist thinking, the premise — the starting point assumption — is incorrect.

Supplement company: We will put the complete list of chemicals into pills and tell people that to ensure their health they should take these pills or powders several times a day to ensure they have all the nutrients they need to be healthy. It is true that many companies do put chemicals in pills and powders. No matter what they call them in marketing, all compounds from any source are chemicals. Some companies actually put laboratory-processed food compounds together under the false assumption that this is somehow better for the body than pills. By the time the faulty reductionist and generalized assumptions reach the supplement company, there is no hope for truth no matter how well-intentioned. It is false assuming that the supplement company will do anything other than hurt your body. It is false to assume that over-replacing any compound is safe. It is false to assume that supplements take the place of natural nutritional food. It is false to assume anything about supplements other than they make those selling them wealthier.

As silly as this all sounds, following false assumptions is precisely what we have been doing in America for over half a century. The matter speaks for itself. Americans are getting sicker and fatter despite ever increasing supplement intake. Supplements are not part of the solution; supplements are increasing the problem.

Drug companies count on your ignorance too

"Let food be thy medicine and medicine be thy food."
—Hippocrates
"Life is like a box of chocolates. " —Forrest Gump

For too many people, their daily pillbox is like the box of chocolates that yielded Tom Hank's memorable quote in *Forrest Gump*. American culture has come to expect a pill for every ache, illness and emotion. Even persons claiming to use natural methods clamor toward processed herbs and unnatural collections and concentrations of vitamins. But first things first.

The first item of business in this chapter is expressing that pharmaceutical companies are not on the whole any different than any other company that sells you things you want to buy. The techniques they use to coerce you into buying follow exactly the same marketing mantra as a car company, shoe company, window company or fragrance/fashion companies: People are stupid and will believe what you tell them if they are either afraid it might be true or they wish it was true. Emotion-driven marketing trumps facts.

Pharmaceutical companies do this to make money just like the other companies. They are not *evil* any more so than any other company turning a profit for their shareholders.

Unlike other companies, drug companies have a low hurdle from compulsion to purchase. It costs very little from your pocket to say yes to their product because someone else is paying for it. Imagine your Air Jordans, Gucci or Tod's only cost a $10 co-pay per pair. You can often go to your physician's office and try the drug company product for free for a week or four. Try that with a hotel room or a car. Unlike other companies, pharmaceutical companies only have to convince you to use their product, not to actually buy it.

However, once you do try it, you have to keep using it indefinitely. While all drugs have side-effects, the majority of patients tolerate the side-effects of one medication fairly well. And that is all the drug company tells you. Many times that is all a physician will tell you.

Although electronic health records (EHRs) are the reason physicians see you with a computer instead of a chart, they do have one very nice attribute: cross checking prescription medications for drug interactions. Other than that, EHRs are a harmful tragedy of wishful socialism politics designed to wrest control of medicine from politically-naïve physicians by promising solutions for non-existent problems — and the topic for another book.

After a few years in practice, most office-based physicians are comfortably rambling off the most likely drug interactions or side-effects a patient can expect based solely upon the chemical class of the drug. Now we can turn the computer screen around and let the patient read pages of drug interactions for their specific pill-popping regimen.

It doesn't make patients feel good about being on the medications, but that is precisely the point. For each medication we give, the body is forced to detoxify one or more chemicals. And we are mucking up the works by perturbing other biochemical reactions that functioned perfectly until we interfered with enzyme function using drugs nature did not intend to be in our body.

If medications didn't interfere with the biochemistry in the body, if medication *only* fixed the one problem for which it is indicated, there would be no side effects. Side-effects do not mean the drug is ineffective — often just the opposite. It is simply that the drug is doing things in your body in addition to what you wanted it to do.

Patients who experience side-effects do one of three things: stop or reduce the drug, suffer through it, or ask their doctor for a different drug with different side effects. In most cases the doctor will comply. Because patients are unaware of side-effects they cannot sense, a doctor may choose a medication that has longer term side-effects to spare the patient short-term discomfort.

When marketing a product, the drug company is going to show you a sad lady on a rainy day taking a pill that turns her into a happy lady on a sunny day. They won't show you that lady in the ER with a hypertensive crisis, bleeding ulcer or simply fifteen pounds fatter. They will show you a happy flitting butterfly landing softly on a sleeping patient's nose and the patient awakening refreshed and smiling (again with the sunny day). They won't show you the patients' blood sugar going up because the sleeping pill worsened the undiagnosed sleep apnea. They won't show you the patient in a car accident because the sleeping pill slowed her reflexes the next day when she'd thought it worn off.

Drug company advertisements will show you white-haired folks frantically scanning for a bathroom due to bladder control issues, then after popping a pill suddenly laughing, doing calisthenics and playing golf while leaving their adult diapers at home. They won't show you those patients living in a nursing home because the medication accelerated dementia. They won't show you the patient in the ER with heat exhaustion. They will show you two people holding hands on the beach (men wouldn't want a pill that makes them cuddle after sex) in adjacent claw-foot bathtubs after presumably exhausting sex reminiscent of their college days. They won't show you the man in the ER with a heart attack or in the oncology ward with malignant melanoma. Nor will they bother to tell you that if the woman takes erectile dysfunction pills she can expect a whopping increase of orgasm sexual pleasure once a month. They won't tell you that erectile dysfunction pills can activate enzymes that cause melanoma skin cancer.

When a chemical has such a complicated course in the body that to know all the reactions a physician would have to do a literature search each year on each of thousands of drugs (we don't), it should be illegal to market that drug directly to consumers. It is impossible for consumers to reasonably know the risks.

Consider this: It is safer to let children smoke cigarettes and drink alcohol than to allow direct to consumer advertising of drugs. Really, kids could always say no to cigarettes, alcohol and drugs too couldn't they? Yet we do not allow children to make this decision. We don't even allow young adults to make this decision. Why? They are not allowed to make that decision because they cannot comprehend all the short and long-term effects. A twenty year-old cannot drink alcohol because they don't comprehend it might land them in the ER or morgue, but a 40 year-old can take numerous pills they cannot possibly comprehend that have the same dangerous effect.

Likewise drug companies will object and state that physicians can always say no, knowing full well that physicians who take hard stands against magic pills lose patients or at a minimum spend unpaid time talking sense into their patients. Drug companies know that physicians who say no lose money one way or the other and thus knowingly place physicians in the only logical position of acceding to their patients and managing the side-effects as they occur. Beyond that, patients can and do get illicit medications from the internet or across U.S. borders. Promising someone magic for free and blaming physicians is not the physician's fault. Nor it is entirely the patient's fault. It is an untenable predicament in which the patient has been promised something that does not exist.

Does that mean drug companies think consumers are stupid or just naïve?

A naïve consumer may believe the first direct to consumer hit. Fool me once, shame on you. Fool me twice, shame on me. No, drug companies know that consumers are stupid. Consumers will believe a thing simply because they wish it to be true.

We are left with another conundrum: Drugs can be useful and necessary. However, drugs can also be re-marketed or developed to treat symptoms of diseases that don't exist or are called syndromes. Some of these syndromes did not exist a few decades ago. Some symptoms do not need to be treated, but consumers can be convinced of insurmountable suffering that must be relieved because no normal person should have these symptoms.

For example, Restless Leg Syndrome (RLS) was invented to market more Parkinson's Disease medications[35]. It worked quite well despite initial physician resistance attributed to what may be medical common sense. The fact is that there is no Parkinson's Disease in the vast majority of these patients. (At least not yet – we can create a brain dependency with these medications however.) In about half of patients diagnosed with RLS, there is *something else* — medications or medical conditions — causing the RLS-like symptoms. What can cause RLS symptoms? Some of the most commonly used medications: those used for allergies and for depression. Alcohol, particularly when used chronically, can damage the liver and cause RLS like symptoms as well[36].

This is called *secondary* RLS and the treatment should be to reverse the *primary* cause (such as medication side-

---

[35] There is a rare genetic disorder than includes RLS. This was described in the 1960s and accounts for less than ten percent of the cases over-diagnosed today.

[36] Franco RA, Ashwathnarayan R, Despandee A. et. al. The High Prevalence of Restless Legs Syndrome Symptoms in Liver Disease in an Academic-Based Hepatology Practice. *J Clin Sleep Med 2008*;4(1):45-49.

effects or iron deficiency). Instead, we provide yet more medication to treat a symptom not the cause. What RLS symptoms suggest is a neurotransmitter imbalance (a deficiency of dopamine) that is most evident when the patient is at rest. The symptom complex wasn't even described until 1960. Yet we did not see a surge in RLS medical literature until the 1990s — strongly suggesting a man-made rather than naturally-occurring condition. Further, we cannot duplicate the symptoms in animals with neurosurgical alteration of animal brains to simulate the proposed brain defect in humans. There are other reasons why the medical community is off-base on RLS, but as this is not a textbook on RLS let us return to the broader picture. What this syndrome suggests is that something in our environment (including food) is disrupting neurotransmitters and some people are more susceptible than others.

Was this disturbance measured objectively? No. And castigation of those trying to help their patients with this symptom complex is not the purpose of this chapter. RLS is only a convenient example — almost *all* chronic conditions are a result of our poisoning our body, mainly by what we put into it.

One recent patient was frustrated with his RLS condition and that the number of pills he was taking had been recently increased by his prior physician, and a prior physician before that also merely added to his pill box. He was very angry that no matter how many pills he took he didn't feel normal. He saw me in consultation because he wanted to try natural (he meant herbal) supplements instead. "Let me get this straight," I said. "You want to try a natural method to normalize your sleep and you'd like to know what herbs and vitamins will do that?"

"Yes! That is exactly it." he smiled.

"Well what could be more natural than not taking any pills at all, herbal or otherwise?"

After some blood tests, I defined a plan to wean him off his over the counter sleeping pill and current herbal supplement, then weaned off his antidepressant while stopping his RLS medication. Three months later, he reported feeling nearly normal. He reported some residual RLS symptoms occurring at the beginning of sleep but no longer awakened him. Reviewing this, we applied a simple method of activating counter-flexors in his legs while falling asleep. In his case, initiating sleep now meant using the covers to pull his feet and toes up toward his head rather than pointed down. He never had symptoms when standing so he simply went to sleep with his leg muscles positioned as if he were standing. Completely cured. He called me two weeks later profusely thankful for the "Dr Frank method" (he coined it for me) and saving him from a lifetime of increasingly toxic pills.

This was just one anecdote and the reader is advised not to self-diagnose simply based upon it. So what about those patients who have conditions not caused by medications?

One could speculate that some food additives that have been linked to behavioral issues in children may also be causing inappropriate nerve imbalance in adults. This would be a brain chemistry issue. Far more encompassing are the chemicals that are not on the food label because legally no disclosure is mandated. The chemicals introduced into food during growth and harvest are present in all conventional food now. Barring a new infectious disease pathogen emerging, no new disease can occur unless it is man-made. It is our prerogative and, indeed, duty to discern what humans have done in the environment to cause new symptoms and symptom complexes to occur. A nearsighted approach would be suppressing the symptom with, in the case of RLS, specific or non-specific brain sedatives or counter-stimulants.

A more commonly and unnecessarily treated symptom is insomnia. Insomnia is not a disease. It is usually not even a condition. It is a normal variation occurring in humans dependent upon a variety of other factors. This does not mean that insomnia, when other symptoms are present as well, cannot be part of an actual disease process but this is the exception.

Sleeping pills, used to treat insomnia, are linked to dementia. It also appears that the more one uses sleeping pills, the stronger the association[37]. Short term use of sleeping pills may be indicated on some occasions. Long term use is not indicated, results in addiction and is associated with increased accidents, especially in women.

Sleeping pills do not restore normal sleep and do not allow restorative sleep. They merely allow patients to pass the night without the frustration of waking up, despite that wakening may be quite normal for some. There are ways to help the body restore this balance without pharmaceutical disruption of the brain's biochemistry. Sometimes the insomnia is worsened by the timing or type of other medications in the body. Sometimes insomnia is caused or worsened by poor dietary, exercise and bedtime habits. The answer should not be to chronically give the body a chemical with toxic effect on numerous receptors in the body that clearly persists into the next day and that are linked to earlier death.

---

[37] S. Billioti de Gage, Y. Moride, T. Ducruet, T. Kurth, H. Verdoux, M. Tournier, A. Pariente, B. Begaud. Benzodiazepine use and risk of Alzheimer's disease: case-control study. *BMJ*, 2014; 349: g5205 DOI: 10.1136/bmj.g5205

Drug companies will not tell you how to cease taking their medicine. Nor frankly, is it their job. However, patients on any pharmaceutical medication chronically may not be doing their job to detoxify their body. The majority of chronic illness requiring medication is due to lifestyle choices. This suggests that most medications can safely be eliminated from the pill box.

Health insurance is not health assurance

"America's health care system is neither healthy, caring, nor a system."
—Walter Cronkite

The main problem with health insurance is that people believe it to be a health care genie: if I or my physician want it, my health insurance should pay for it. Health insurance should be thought of as disease management insurance. Health insurance manages your diseases, it does not manage your health.

While I do enjoy political discussions in real life, this chapter will only discuss the reality of medical insurance and how individuals must modify their perception of their health insurance to achieve health assurance. With one brief exception regarding preventative care, I'll refrain from the political.

Health insurance, like any insurance, is a contract of risk. In exchange for money, a company agrees to pay for specified items *if* they occur. For any insurance company to stay in business, it must take more money from patients than it pays out to patients. Therefore, the majority of people MUST pay more in than they get back — just like any other insurance.

Health insurance is like car insurance. It helps pay for broken things. Your car insurance does not pay for regular maintenance. It doesn't pay for gas, oil, windshield wiper fluid or car washes. It doesn't pay for new tires although it will give your car transportation to the shop in an accident. If something bad happens to your car, you pay the agreed to deductible and your insurance pays what they agreed to. The amount you and your insurance pay to fix your car depends upon what coverage you chose to purchase. You don't have to have car insurance, but if government officials catch you without car insurance, you will pay a fine.

Health insurance is similar to house insurance. Your house insurance doesn't pay for the monthly prescriptions for cable, gas, electric or water. Your house insurance doesn't pay for the maintenance needed to keep the house in shape and healthy. If your roof starts deteriorating because you didn't maintain it, your insurance does not pay for a new roof. However, if your house is traumatized by an accident, someone purposefully hurts your house or its contents, or it catches fire and is damaged even if it is because you didn't do your best to prevent these things, your insurance pays what it agreed to and you pay the deductible dependent upon what coverage you chose to purchase.

Health insurance, like other insurances, does not assure your health, just as life insurance doesn't assure your life. Life insurance pays when you lose your life; health insurance pays when you lose your health.

Health insurance does not pay to keep you healthy (the exception being certain preventative care mandates in the Affordable Care Act, like vaccines and some disease screening like colonoscopy for colon cancer prevention). It does not pay for anything other than what you agreed to in your policy. It does not pay for a therapy simply because you or your physician think it is necessary. It does not pay for what you want. It pays for what it thinks you need for the given diagnosis, which is determined by the policy you signed.

A physician has two choices: recommend the best treatment course or recommend a course the insurance will pay for. Generally, insurance will pay for the least expensive option which — unless there is a definitive cure — is designed to improve symptoms (how a patient feels) but not correct the problem. About 10% of patients will choose the curative route if not paid for by insurance.

It is a rare patient that chooses the inexpensive option then refrains from complaining about how they want the best treatment but can't afford it. What they mean is they want the most expensive treatment but don't want to reprioritize to afford it. You cannot assure your health by relying on your insurance. You cannot assure your health by waiting for someone to pay your way. You can only assure your health by making the most healthful choices every day.

For chronic conditions (those lasting more than a few weeks), the best treatment course is not covered by insurance at all. For chronic conditions, the best treatment is to eliminate the cause of the symptoms rather than merely reducing the symptoms themselves. The best treatment course, the only way to get well and stay well, the only way to stop being sick, fat and tired, is to regain your health.

That means patients need to do something other than pop a pill or take a shot. Your health insurance company is not supposed to care about you. They are supposed to pay for what you agreed to in your contract with them. You are supposed to care about you. Your physician cares about you but is not supposed to pay for you. You are supposed to pay for you. Too often patients would rather get angry with some faceless company instead of getting angry with the face they see in the mirror and take charge of their health by actively doing something about their health.

There is nothing more miserable than a patient who feels sorry for herself and refuses to doing anything to help herself. It is yet more annoying to have a patient who "cannot afford" the chiropractor, the yoga classes, the therapist, the fresh vegetables but still smokes cigarettes, drinks martinis and eats at restaurants each week.

Health insurance is not your mother. It doesn't care if you make stupid choices. It won't change what you agreed to in your insurance contract. Unlike your mother, the health insurance company will feel no pain in punishing you in the form of higher premium increases each year you have poor choices registered in your health record. Further, poor lifestyle choices that lead to increasing health insurance premiums now frequently increase your car and life insurance premiums as well.

Your physicians are not paid to counsel you on a healthy diet and weight loss. When you hear advice about changing your lifestyle choices, you are hearing someone who cares about you enough to give their time to you without being paid for it even though they could be making money writing prescriptions for someone else. That will not change. As health insurance, medications and procedures get more expensive, there is less money to pay for people's time.

What should you do as the person who cares most about your body? Honestly discuss with your physician how you can treat the CAUSE of your symptoms and be willing to pay for that treatment with your time and your finances.

If your car won't run correctly because you've been feeding it low octane gas and your mechanic tells you it must have high octane gas, you can either feed your car what it needs (costing you more long-term for gas for the life of your car) or he can tow your car from the shop to work, solving your short-term problem. After all, towing your car is free. It is covered by your insurance. Gas is not free. You'd actually have to give up something else to feed your car properly so that it can run properly.

If your lower back won't run correctly because you've been feeding it the wrong food, your physician can give you some pills to get you to work (after all, the insurance pays for the pills), or you can eat the right foods in the right amount to correct the obesity that caused your pain after a chiropractor re-aligns you.

Like your car and your house, the way to keep your body in optimal shape is to daily make the right decisions that often involve some time and planning and always involves keeping the body in optimal shape for as long as the body is designed to exist. None of those decisions are supported by your insurance nor should they be. Insurance is for catastrophic events that hopefully will happen very rarely.

When faced with poor health, the very last question you ask should be: how can I re-arrange my life to pay for it? Many times, eliminating the unhealthful choices (alcohol, tobacco, supplements, processed foods, restaurant food, improper portions) more than pays for the new health changes. In some instances — such as tobacco and fat elimination — you may even pay less for health, car and life insurance.

Fat isn't simple arithmetic

"An ounce of prevention is worth a pound of cure."

—Benjamin Franklin

"Every human being is the author of his own health or disease."

—Gautama Buddha

Many people poorly understand nutrition and body composition. This lack of understanding includes physicians and other health care providers. Included in this lack of understanding is the false premise that a calorie is a calorie. This is, in essence, what physicians are taught and frankly in an inpatient hospital setting or in an analytical laboratory this premise serves in calculating and maintaining patients *temporarily* when they cannot consume food through normal means for whatever reason.

This premise fails miserably, however, when dealing with outpatients and chronic illness, such as obesity. If it worked, treating obesity would be much easier. Indeed, equating a calorie in one person as having the same effect in another is analogous to saying a standard octane gallon of gas will cause a Prius, a Suburban SUV and a Mercedes Coup all to function the same for the same distance. Compared to human beings, cars are simple machines with barely any variability or complexity. So if a standard unit of energy does not produce the same result in a simple machine, why would we expect a standard unit of energy to produce the same result in the complexity of humans? Yet we physicians disbelieve our patients when they tell us this about their bodies.

The biochemical pathways in one cell alone are impossible for us to duplicate. We cannot even accurately map all these reactions in an interactive bio-simulation manner with a computer. Consider then how any given unit of food energy — a calorie — may function differently not only between persons but also in the same person throughout the course of a day, in the context of stress, illness, pregnancy, menstruation, sleep, activity and aging. It is also why patients get frustrated when they try a weight loss program or fitness program that works for a friend but not for them.

At least once a week I will have a patient in my office crying about her inability to lose weight. She'll think something's wrong with her (other than the weight), and it doesn't help that society vacillates between fat-teasing (which helps no one) and fat celebration (which started by telling obese patients they could stay obese and be healthy). No one can be fat and healthy.

If fat functioned metabolically exactly like muscle, there would be no health problem associated with fat, it would be a purely cosmetic concern.

It is not simply a cosmetic concern; fat makes you sick and tired. And despite decades of empty promises from supplement companies, drug companies, cosmetic companies, spa treatments and diet gurus, NOTHING has stopped this trend toward misery and earlier death.

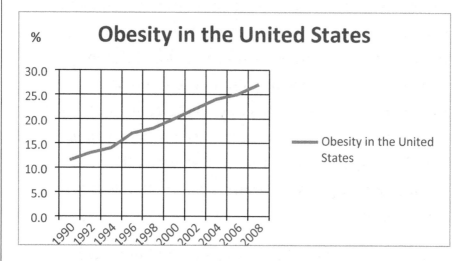

Data from NHANES and www.data360.org

While the graph stops at 2008, be assured that in the United States obesity is now above thirty percent. This is the tip of the iceberg. Feeding the fat are persons of all ages, and now even children are being sentenced to a miserable life mainly by what they are fed. The number of overweight persons is twice the obese number.

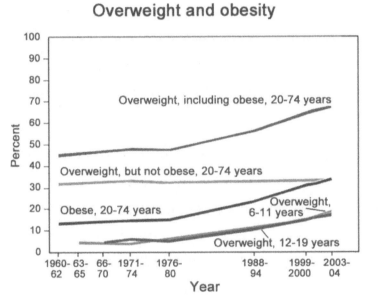

Overweight and obesity

SOURCES: Centers for Disease Control and Prevention, National Center for Health Statistics, Health, United States, 2006, Figure 13. Data from the National Health and National Examination Survey.

These data are from public government sources, telling us that not only is the government well-aware of the problem but also that this worsening problem is not secret information. The source of this problem will be covered later in the book.

For the balance of this chapter, let us simply return to our fat discussion. Obesity cannot be resolved by treating fat. Fat is the symptom, not the disease.

Obesity can be corrected in one of two ways. By either normalizing the metabolism or surgically removing the stomach and re-routing the intestines. Given that about 2% of patients will die from the latter and the survivors will spend their remaining life hating food, surgery should only be a recommendation for a highly-select group of patients. Less extreme surgical options are not nearly as effective, reinforce unhealthy eating habits and have little chance of addressing the chronic underlying metabolic dysfunction.

Patients first need to understand that some fat is healthy — both on their bodies and in their food. Just as there are important (essential) amino acids, there are important (essential) fats. A standard energy unit in the body is called a calorie. The body is designed to efficiently store any extra calories as fat because our ancestors lived at a time where excess food was rare rather than a daily occurrence. We also inherited strong protections against getting too thin. Whenever we eat until we are full, we will create fat.

When patients lose fat, they will not get too thin. However, they may be told they look too thin, sick or old due to loss of subcutaneous fat tissue. This is the fat directly beneath the skin. This is more prominent in women due to a greater amount of subcutaneous fat and thinner skin. The fat loss, particularly in the face and upper body, does not mean the body has lost too much fat. When enough fat is lost, previously stretched skin sags or wrinkles appear for the same reason. That is a result of being obese too long, not from now being thin. Understanding this, and that the skin will partially compensate — eventually, is important to help anticipate the negative emotions which might otherwise demotivate patients.

The healthiest fat is the type that regulates temperature. This type of fat is called brown fat and helps protect the spine and some organs. The least healthy fat is storage fat, particularly around the abdomen, which appears white in most microscopic slides but yellow during surgery. Storage fat is meant to be very temporary and when used that way is not unhealthy. Nature likes big butts not big guts.

As previously discussed, our ancient ancestors, whose genes are now our genes, consumed essential fats (the omega-6 and omega-3 fats) in 1:1 ratio that we know naturally occurred in their diet of free-range meat[38], fish, plants[39], nuts and fruit.[40] In contrast, Americans consume

---

[38] n-3 Fatty Acids in Eggs from Range-Fed Greek Chickens. N Engl J Med. 1989;321(20):1412-1412.

over ten times the amount of omega-6 compared to omega-3, an inflammatory ratio that our genetic heritage does not accommodate[41].

As of 2012, about half of all U.S. adults — 117million people — had one or more chronic health conditions, such as obesity, heart disease, cancer and diabetes[42]. About eighty percent of these chronic health conditions directly result from diet and environment choices. The huge number of impacted people leaves little doubt that the types of fat we eat daily is most seriously affecting us.

The highest sources of omega-6 in our diet come from common oils: corn oil, soy oil, canola oil, safflower oil. These are found in almost every condiment, dessert and processed baked good. Compounding the inflammation are the chemists who hydrogenate the oils in the lab, turning unsaturated oils into saturated oils. This makes vegetable oil taste like animal fat and gives the oil longer shelf-life before becoming rancid. The price is paid by the consumer's health. The ratio of saturated fats increase

---

[39] Robinson F. Power-Packed Purslane. Mother Earth News. April/May 2005.
[40] Simonpoulos AP. Omega-3 fatty acids and antioxidants in edible wild plants, nuts and seeds Asia Pac journal of Clin Nutrition. 2002. Doi: 10.1111/ajc.2002.11.issue-s6/issuetoc.

[41] Van Vleit T, Katan MB. Lower ratio of n-3 to n-6 fatty acids in cultured than in wild fish. Am J Cin Nutr 1990.
[42] Ward BW, Schiller JS, Goodman RA. Multiple chronic conditions among US adults: a 2012 update. Prev Chronic Dis. 2014;11:130389. DOI: http://dx.doi.org/10.5888/pcd11.130389.

and the double bonds that are disturbed will form both "cis" and "trans". (For a quick review, revisit the "How Fats and Oils are Named" located in the Conventional Foods chapter.)

The schematic below shows the standard representation of chemical bonds. By convention, a single bond is a single line (—) whereas a double bond is a double line (=).

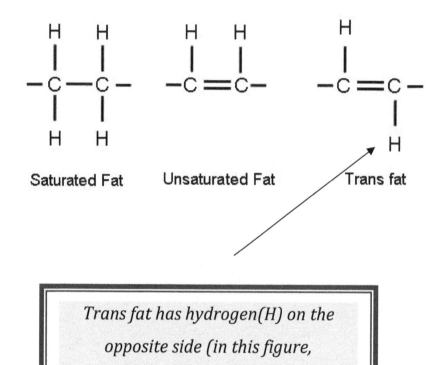

Saturated Fat   Unsaturated Fat   Trans fat

> *Trans fat has hydrogen(H) on the opposite side (in this figure, downward)*

Cis bonds are common in nature; trans bonds are much less common. Additionally the trans bonds that form during laboratory processing are not in the position in the molecule that exist naturally. Remember that enzymes are like a lock and key: if the key is changed slightly it will not open the lock. Thus, enzymes that manage a cis bond cannot process a trans bond. Despite having the same elemental chemistry, the stereoisomer (a three-dimensional form) is completely different. For an analogy, let's look at a piece of paper. You can fold it into a paper airplane or crumple it into a ball, a completely different three-dimensional form composed of exactly the same thing.

We accelerated heart disease in an entire generation by pushing margarine (hydrogenated oil) into our diets replacing butter — with perhaps the exception of Wisconsin which resisted the margarine craze until 1967. If you think it's butter, but it's not, you probably have some stents in your arteries if you are still alive. It took us decades to uncover and address this to the unsuspecting public and stands as a warning beacon whenever any government agency or guideline is pushed upon us. Physicians are taught very little biochemistry. Even so, we owe the American public a huge mea culpa for not pushing for long-term safety data, and this may also be why some physicians are now willing to break ranks on important public health topics government agencies refuse to adequately address. Chronic diseases and conditions are the most common, costly, and preventable of all health problems. Yet we have not prevented them[43].

Back to real fats and oils. We also get the inflammatory omega-6 oils in farm-raised animals (beef, pork, chickens and fish) as previously discussed. It is important to realize that after weaning, humans can get all essential fats from plants. We do not need animals, their eggs or their udder secretions to satisfy our essential fatty acid needs. We also do not need animals or their products to satisfy our protein needs. But we do need a variety of plant types to satisfy the necessary protein components called amino acids — which vegans successfully demonstrate.

The next point of educating patients is also simple: if you want to get rid of unhealthy and unneeded fat, stop eating the unhealthy and unneeded fat. While this point is simple, the application is not as easy. For example, a moderately obese person 30 – 40 pounds overweight can easily live two months on that fat alone. Depending upon the body size and activity level, a pound of fat can power the body for 1 – 3 days. Knowing this, physicians can reliably advise patients than any program advertising losing inches (or dress sizes) in hours or several pounds overnight are merely temporarily moving water around, not fat.

---

[43] http://www.cdc.gov/chronicdisease/overview/index.htm

Our ancestors also gave us a liking for the taste of fat, which for them was a survival mechanism powering their body through leaner times and ensuring reproduction. Overly thin women are not as fertile and are poor vessels for a fetus. Thin men were at a competitive disadvantage despite the fact that lean mass increases testosterone. Babies like fat, a liking that is satisfied with breast milk from birth. Lean mothers do not yield as much fat in breast milk, making baby survival less likely.

Fat is calorie dense. A mouthful of fat gives the body four times more energy than a mouthful of potato. The types of essential fats in human milk is very different than those found in cow's milk and contains some fats necessary for brain development not found in cow milk. In addition, cow milk has far more calcium— up to three times more — than does human milk. Evolutionarily it makes sense for cows. Why would any animal make breast milk suboptimal for its offspring? The offspring would be likely to die and not reproduce the next generation; that animal species would become extinct.

Consider again at the periodic table of the elements[44]. What might be wrong with too much calcium (Ca)? It will compete with similarly shaped and charged elements such

---

[44] http://webelements.com/

as magnesium (Mg) and possibly other similarly-charged elements, such as iron (Fe) and zinc (Zn). Cow's milk has too much calcium for human babies. What do we know about babies fed cow's milk instead of human milk? They have weaker immune systems. Iron and zinc are necessary components for the immune system.

Remember, more than the body needs is usually as bad as not enough. A large amount of non-human dairy in the diet after weaning is not balanced. The balanced amount of fat, calcium and micronutrients in breast milk is designed by ancestral genes to meet the needs of a growing infant for two to three years. No milk is designed to meet the needs of an adult but may still be part of a balanced organic diet. In terms of diet, milk would have been used in a fermented (cultured) form. To ferment dairy, the dairy product is first digested by bacteria. The bacteria used are the same type that our ancient ancestors discovered and used to ferment dairy to produce yoghurt, kefir and cheese. The bacteria and human digestive system were compatible – the bacteria would be eaten along with the dairy and but did not cause disease in the human. In exchange, the human gut provided a warm safe environment for the bacteria to thrive. These harmless bacteria used the resources that harmful bacteria would have needed to survive. The harmless bacteria also created waste products that discouraged harmful bacteria and other harmful organisms. Biology calls this a symbiotic relationship: two species (human and bacteria) mutually benefit each other.

Where does that leave dairy in terms of fat? Dairy must follow the philosophy of eating what our ancient genes expect in a manner that still allows us to function in modern society.

What does this look like for the average person? Choosing organic grass-fed dairy from cows and goats, particularly from dairy that is fermented. Avoiding artificially separated dairy by using whole milk and milk fat. The bulk of milk fat (cream) will float to the top naturally, but skimmed milk (zero percent fat milk) would not have been part of ancient humans' diets. Avoid regular consumption of mammal flesh (particularly any hoofed animal).

Why the restrictions? Skimmed milk was not in your ancestors' diets; conventional red meat is unhealthy and wild game is not an option for most people.

More on breast milk

Breast milk from the mother is the perfect nutrition for any infant mammal, which includes humans. There is no synthetic substitute that nourishes and protects infants better than breast milk. Breastfeeding strengthens the maternal bond, provides passive immunity to the infant for diseases the mother has already survived and requires no special pasteurization or disinfection methods to protect the infant. Breastfed infants have lifelong lower incidence of immune system disorders – less asthma and less leukemia for example. So valuable is breast milk to infants that in countries without safe water supply, medical experts recommend breastfeeding even if the mother is infected with HIV (which can be passed in breast milk). Nursing mothers also benefit. Breastfeeding is protective against breast cancer and nursing mothers are more likely to return to their pre-pregnancy body weight and less likely to develop diabetes.

When fish and flesh were previously discussed, the data showed that the healthiest non-toxic sources were wild or grass-fed without any exposure to man-made chemicals. This leaves one remaining source of fat — plants.

Plant oils, including nut oils, can be healthier sources of essential fatty acids. Because many man-made toxins are lipophilic (fat-loving), the toxins easily accumulate not only in animal fats but also in plant oils. For this reason, plant oils can also have high levels of toxins. Toxins in the soil or sprayed on the plant will concentrate in the fat soluble oils of the plant. Toxins on the equipment used to harvest and process the plant can dissolve in the plant oils and any fat-soluble substance containing collected plant oils can also dissolve into the oil. Oils exposed to air will oxidize (become rancid) over time, adding toxins to a previously healthy collection.

Oil dissolves fat-soluble products. Storing oil in plastic or plastic-coated metal is not the best choice. Chemists store chemicals in glass, the most inert form of container to avoid this type of contamination.

Choose glass bottles for your oils and fats. Choose glass bottles for your dairy when possible. If you cannot purchase in glass containers, you can minimize the surface contact area to volume slightly by buying very large containers, keeping the container away from heat and light, or by transferring the contents to a glass or ceramic container. Minimizing the air contact with the oil will also preserve the oil from turning rancid as quickly. Some may choose kiln-glazed ceramic as containers to reduce light exposure. Remember to be forward-thinking and reuse or recycle glass.

To recapitulate, why the long discussion about fats and oils? Because it has a huge impact upon your health.

Abdominal fat is unhealthy and promotes inflammation. People with excess abdominal fat can expect to be sicker, in more pain and have shorter lives. Losing unwanted abdominal fat and keeping it off cannot be done unless normal body chemistry is restored. Remember: no more poisoned plate, poisoned water and poison pills. It takes about two hours in my clinic to define a personalized program ensuring patients' successful weight loss.

The basic steps for any program are in this book, and every patient that adheres to it loses their excess fat. Due to demand by early reviewers of this text, an accompanying workbook and web application are in development to provide the antidote for your poisoned plate.

Take Medical Organizations with a Grain of Salt

"No, no, you're not thinking; you're just being logical."

—Niels Bohr

The main problem with medical association guidelines is that we believe them more than what they are. Medical guidelines are uneasy agreements among politically-motivated persons much learned in one small area of human health who digest huge amounts of data and then throw it up onto beleaguered colleagues and the unsuspecting public. Guidelines are always compromises by thought leaders or political leaders in a particular medical specialty. Data published by persons serving on the medical guideline committee is always over-represented, particularly if the recommendation involves a drug or device for which the thought leader was paid, by the pharmaceutical company, to represent. Study data from products without strong financial backing is generally ignored. When physicians read these guidelines, we are often displeased but somewhat bound: ignoring medical guidelines presents legal risks to physicians even if the guidelines were not appropriate for a particular patient.

Despite all this, there is little better from which to guide patient treatment, and there are far worse alternatives which are discussed primarily in the government guidelines chapter. What will not be specifically discussed is the wide swath of pseudo-providers who, for various motivations, pass off marketing data as real and in the process harm their patients (albeit unknowingly or at least uncaringly). The other problem is with the patients themselves. Patients will assume that all data by those who call themselves health providers is valid. It is not.

When patients assume all healthcare providers have equivalent medical knowledge, regardless of the degree or letters behind the professional's name, the patient will not think for themselves. With that often erroneous assumption of trust, the patient may conclude that taking this herb, taking this "special" vitamin, "special" mineral, extract of whombatwonk kernals (fictitious), drinking this specially-ionized water, applying proprietary detoxifying tape to their feet... can cure their cancer, fatigue, hair loss, wrinkles, acne, ulcers, obesity, diabetes. The patient then misses an opportunity to slow or stop their disease with a proven treatment using the scientific method. Without a factual premise, the conclusion is unreliable.

Thus, THE MAJORITY OF WHAT AMERICANS DO TO IMPROVE THEIR HEALTH IS UNRELIABLE AND SOMETIMES DANGEROUS.

There is a reason the scientific method is called scientific. This method is the only way to use facts to discover more facts. There are some schools of health care that derive treatment protocols from the scientific method. The rest do not. The rest use marketing tools, such as word-of-mouth and misleading advertising, which are only case reports at best. In layman's terms, a case report is an anecdote. A medical anecdote is a bit like the stories you hear in the high school locker room with about half as much truthfulness.

This doesn't mean case reports are not useful. But appropriate use is jogging physician minds out of complacency and to consider a new possibility. As in: *Hmm, this patient's case showed an unusual reaction to a medication while he also had this rare medical condition. Perhaps we should do a literature search for similar cases.* A case report can eventually can lead to a randomized controlled trial that can give us true cause and effect with a professional statistician or more often disprove the new possibility entirely but in a scientifically sound manner.

A case report is an anecdote. It may be completely off-base and usually is. A case report should never be used to raise treatment expectations; it should be used to raise eyebrows — of physician researchers.

However, if someone is selling a product that is not submitted to the Food and Drug Administration (FDA), the case report can legally be used for marketing the product and the patients will never know the difference. That is, after all, the first rule of marketing: people are stupid, they will believe a thing because they simply wish it to be true. My mantra: God is the only one I'll trust without statistically significant data. Everything else is simply an opinion.

With a case report (or if the quack wants to be extremely impressive, a compilation of case reports — which has about as much statistical worth as a single case report — *none*) one can fashion a "medical" or "health" newsletter and exclaim, "Joe Smith tried years of traditional therapy for Xerxses Disease without success, but after just 30 days on Dr. Frank's Wonder Elixir from fresh elk horn velvet rubbed off on birch trees and the proprietary blend of swamp herbs and civet cat droppings, not only did Joe Smith's snoring disappear but it cured his baldness and he can pleasure his wife in bed for hours!"

(Joe Smith is fictitious. So is his wife, but she bought all the elixir regardless so don't write me for more.)

Never believe a testimonial.

Never believe a testimonial.

Never believe a testimonial.

As a general rule for lay persons, do not believe any product study unless it involves a minimum of 100 patients, use a "case control" design (which will be in the study description), utilizes at least three geographically and financially distinct sites, and is either audited by an independent company OR is not paid for by the company who profits from the product being studied.

The greatest benefit of medical organization's clinical recommendations is protecting patients from misleading marketing data. Because science-based medical organizations know the hucksterism occurs, they offer a unified front for consistent clinical approaches. This usually involves analysis and consensus opinion on scientifically-run studies. If the general population had the ability to do this, there would be no purpose for medical organizations offering recommendations and guidelines.

In short, physicians are human and do humane service for their profession as well as to the broader population with clinical practice guidelines. These guidelines provide consistency and ease of application to patients. Three common medical organizations are the American College of Physicians, American College of Obstetrics and Gynecology and the American College of Surgeons.

It isn't a perfect system. Physicians are human and foster prideful and sometimes greedy actions in consensus, particularly if the goal is publication or other public accolades[45]. Consensus means not all physicians agreed with the recommended approaches. Further, if a physician brings a fresh approach, no matter how logical, academics will destroy the upstart[46] — so never expect momentous breakthroughs. Medical consensus is slow to change. This means newer clinical data is often not incorporated. And politics can taint the recommendations. The taint can occur due to personal bias which was rampant in HIV testing and treatment guidelines and quite evident whenever huge profits are involved. This is occurring in HPV testing and vaccination for cervical cancer as well as with Hepatitis C treatments.

Recommendations can also be tainted when physicians are strong-armed into adopting politically-driven recommendations. Most visible to patients would be the forcible ejection of "old fashioned medicine" in favor of computerized medical records — Electronic Medical Records (EHR). This single cave-in by medicine allowed the government — not your physician — to dictate your medical care by letting the government decide what a physician must do in order to receive payment. This gradual erosion means eventually neither you nor your

[45] Haug CJ. Peer-Review Freaud — Hacking the Scientific Publication Process. NEJM 373:25. 2393-95. DOi 10.1056/NEJMMp1512330
[46] Gonzalez NJ, Isaacs LL. The Trophoblast and the Origins of Cancer. One solution to the medical enigma of our time. 2009. New Spring Press. NY NY.

physician will decide what is best for you. The government will decide, particularly after 2019 when physicians must provide the government your personal information in order to get paid.

So with all the problems, why should we bother with medical organization recommendations?

Despite these disclaimers and examples, physician groups tend toward caution with recommendations. We wish to maintain public trust as contemplative protectors. If group consensus changed dramatically with every research study, the guidelines would be little better than the marketing hucksters that simply want to sell a product. From the standpoint of both education and skill, no one can better advise you regarding safety, effectiveness and personal appropriateness of a treatment approach than can a physician skilled in research methods. However, there are very few such physicians in clinical practice and even fewer who have the time to digest and incorporate research advances. This leaves most patients with the next best thing: physicians using recommendations found in medical consensus groups. These drive the clinical practice guidelines that can be used by any physician.

Simply stated, be informed, but also be informed from whence comes your information. Find a physician comfortable disclosing to you that there is some disagreement by the experts on various topics. Learn the difference between data and marketing or you can never make informed decisions about your health.

Government Guidelines: Weak Science, Unintended Consequences

"The greatest advances of civilization, whether in architecture or painting, in science and literature, in industry or agriculture, have never come from centralized government." —Milton Friedman

"A collection of a hundred Great brains makes one big fathead." —Carl Jung

"A collection of thousands of mediocre brains makes one big government."

—Dr Frank

If science by consensus is fraught with legitimate concern, then government guidelines by consensus is a mess of mediocrity guaranteed to harm those governed.

In medicine, we have some conciliation that those forming guidelines are among the most learned and, at least, have been taught to and taken an oath to "first do no harm." In contrast, the government cares little about us as individuals. Anyone who has had the misfortune to interact with any government agency can attest to this.

While many public officials may be said to have good intentions, that paved road leads nowhere good. You can't vote out unelected government workers, and the vast majority of the government is precisely that: unanswerable to you in any way and worse, able to force its policies into your personal life.

With that background, how can we expect anything but harm to come from government guidelines and mandates? The examples chosen for this book have a common theme: A failure of government and government scientists to wait for solid prospective safety evidence before artificially changing our food and water supply.

 Harm, when it involves health, is exactly what the government has historically given. That is simply expected when whole government institutions are driven to produce something, anything, to justify their existence in state and federal budget line items. Further, no individual is held responsible for anything. Compounding that are politicians threatening departmental budget cuts if the guidelines are harmful to their political backers, such as conventional food manufacturers, chemical companies and manufacturing unions.

Government officials making the health care decisions for the collective nation do not have data or the expertise required to ensure sound decisions. Uninformed decisions — and all political decisions regarding health are at best misinformed — not only fail to protect but often harm the public. The few officials that have credentials lack accountability for their repeated failures. As stated earlier, you cannot vote out unelected public officials. The common thread in all government policy errors is acting based upon belief and conjecture rather than upon complete and valid data.

Prohibition: Religious zealots in government run rampant

Historically, the U.S. government's first big step into public health came with the Prohibition movement beginning in the 1830s. The government had run out of emotionally charged wars against England and had to placate voters by fueling the fire of those who believed many social evils stemmed from alcohol. Maine and Oregon enacted legislation first, prohibiting the manufacture and sale of alcohol by 1847, and Protestant (Methodists specifically) beliefs fueled formation of political Temperance Unions, furthering their goal of enforced alcohol abstinence. Where this belief was resisted, coercion and outright vandalism and violence occurred, best characterized by Carrie Nation's antics. That her first husband died from alcoholism did not dissuade her, for as always, political integrity is an oxymoron.

Several states followed with prohibition laws, totaling thirteen states by 1855.

The United States was distracted from this debacle briefly with the Civil War, but not even the emotional drain of this horrendous tragedy was sufficient pause for reflection. This trend could have been informative had the government in those states actually analyzed the crime data. Instead, the government used the histrionics of religious leaders to fuel elections and votes.

In 1919, the 18th amendment to the U.S. Constitution made alcohol illegal and remained so until 1933 when the 21st amendment repealed the 18th and alcohol again became legal.

For one hundred years, various areas of the United States were subjected to unsubstantiated religious fervor turned into laws. Further, both the process and the laws led to unnecessary violence against those with opposing views and, in the case of Women's Christian Temperance Union leader Frances Willard, violence directed toward black men and recommendations that black men who drink alcohol should be lynched — scapegoating black men as a threat to white women.

This tragedy could have been avoided if government officials had simply applied logic rather than fear. Instead, the government learned that if it could appease irrational citizens, their careers in government would be strongly reinforced. Damage done by the government is long-lasting and sometimes irreparable: Michigan is still dealing with the heavy-handed liquor tax from the Prohibition era in 2015 — a tax that stifles growth and depresses wages.[47]

Working up to an amendment took decades and coordination. No votes are needed, however, to pass government guidelines and modify regulations in the name of public health. The danger of national agencies and institutes is that they can inflict unintentional harm on the entire nation without any voter recourse or consent.

Fluoride: If a little is good, a lot must be better

Fluoride is touted as a crowning achievement in public health by public health officials. Unfortunately this mediocrity probably is the crowning achievement of public health despite the harm known to result from poor implementation and an abject failure of quality control, the long-term effects of which is now becoming increasingly apparent.

Lauding its own accomplishment, the U.S. Centers for Disease Control and Prevention state "Fluoridation of community drinking water is a major factor responsible

---

[47] http://www.detroitnews.com/story/opinion/editorials/2015/10/03/editorial-lighten-prohibition-era-taxes-craft-liquor

for the decline in dental caries (tooth decay) during the second half of the 20th century. The history of water fluoridation is a classic example of clinical observation leading to epidemiologic investigation and community-based public health intervention. Although other fluoride-containing products are available, water fluoridation remains the most equitable and cost-effective method of delivering fluoride to all members of most communities, regardless of age, educational attainment, or income level."[48] Data supports this public health statement.

However, nowhere does the data support this question: is fluoride *needed* to prevent tooth decay? The answer is "no." Fluoride is unnecessary. We shall explore this more with dental data from around the world.

Objectively, fluoridation of the public water supplies did appear to deliver the intended outcome: fewer dental cavities. This health achievement should not be belittled — but not because people need fluoride to have healthy teeth. Better oral hygiene improved health because persons who choose to not use proper oral hygiene *and* do not have fluoridated water will lose their teeth more quickly and have overall worse health as a result of the inflammation and infections that can occur with poor dental hygiene. At the time the government pushed fluoride into our drinking water, however, there was no

[48] MMWR Weekly. October 22, 1999 /48(41);933-940.

medical evidence to indicate benefits beyond control of cavities. Dental cavities is not a "disease" per se, but rather a condition resulting from unhealthful individual choices.

So what happened to countries that did NOT fluoridate their water?

These trend lines graphed for the World Health Organization (WHO) compiled by Malmö University, Sweden in 2012 compare countries where water or salt was fluoridated compared with non-fluoridated countries.

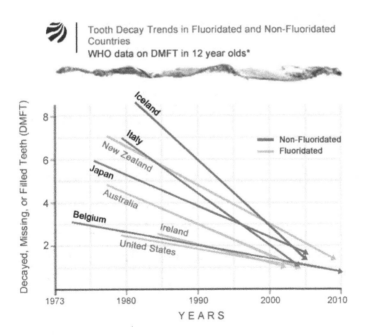

Tooth Decay Trends in Fluoridated and Non-Fluoridated Countries
WHO data on DMFT in 12 year olds*

What the U.S. health policy czars didn't ask was : is fluoride needed? Clearly not.

The World Health Organization showed us that countries *without* fluoride decreased cavities at least as well as the United States and *all* countries showed a decline in cavities regardless of whether or not they were fluoridated. Logically this is most likely due to education about oral hygiene and improved dentistry. In fact, several countries *without* fluoride reduced dental decay *faster* than did the United States.

Biochemically, there is no doubt that fluoride applied to tooth enamel increases resistance to tooth decay. Fluoride in tiny concentrations is not harmful to tooth structure, provides resistance to decay and can, at higher concentrations, cause unsightly permanent cosmetic changes in the tooth enamel ranging from white spots to brown discoloration. This observation was noted in the early 1900s in Colorado and made known by Dr. Frederick McKay, a dentist, after being reported earlier in Germany by Dr. Carl Erhardt in the 1870s. By 1940, Michigan initiated a prospective observation of children in Grand Rapids, where fluoride had been introduced into the water supply. Over those fifteen years, the tooth decay in Grand Rapids children diminished rapidly.

This public health observation was used as proof to begin public water fluoridation throughout the nation in the

1960s such that the majority of Americans were exposed by 2000. The assumption by all early researchers was that fluoride had to be taken internally to strengthen the teeth, despite that groups of dentists were actively applying high concentrations of fluoride gels to teeth in the 1970s, a practice that should have caused serious contemplation in the government agencies. It did not.

Unfortunately, fluoride was America's first failure of the "super-size me" approach to all things. The first mistake was the assumption that fluoride needed to be taken internally. It does not, but this was ignored prior to adding fluoride to public water. The second mistake was believing that the high concentrations of fluoride used would be safe and effective. It is not. The third mistake was exposing very young children to fluoride prior to their teeth erupting — providing little benefit yet risking fluorosis — permanent changes to the cosmetic and, rarely, structure of the teeth and weakening of bones.

The benefit of fluoride in preventing tooth decay occurs by exposing tooth enamel to very low levels of fluoride over time. This makes the teeth more resistant to acid and helps inhibit some of the bacteria enzymes that live in the plaque around the teeth and gums. This low level can be easily achieved with quantifiable amounts of toothpaste to which fluoride has been added. It is completely unnecessary to add fluoride to the water to which everyone is unwillingly exposed, everyone including both infants and elderly who can only be harmed.

In high concentrations, fluoride can weaken bones, disrupt calcium metabolism and interfere with thyroid function. Fluoride competes with Iodine, the latter being much more critical to proper function of the body metabolism than pretty teeth[49]. This is simply the fluoride biochemistry. We will not see a fifteen year study of an entire city to examine fluoride harm for numerous reasons, but at the core, public health agencies will not promote studies revealing the idiocracy of public health institutions. While such studies are mandated by the government for private industries (such as drug companies and factories), the government will never hold its own agencies to the same scrutiny to which it holds private citizens.

The government states that its biggest challenge to fluoridation are unsubstantiated claims of adverse health effects. The truth is that the biggest challenge is substantiated: there is no long-term safety data on fluoride at various concentrations and the natural history of over-fluoridation around the world indicates probable harm. Also substantiated are data from countries other than the United States showing better dental health in

---

[49] Brownstein D. Overcoming Thyroid Disorders. Third Ed. Medical Alternative Press. 2014. West Bloomfield MI.

countries with no fluoride. In other words the U.S. public health service blew it, and any future directives from public health should be heavily scrutinized. Lack of data does not mean safe as the U.S. government's FDA tells pharmaceutical and medical device companies all the time. Any regulation the government does not apply to itself will hurt the public.

Margarine — Chemists breaking our hearts

"Margarine" is a category of fake butters. Historically margarine is a moving target worth exploring to better understand how harmful margarines came to market.

Margarine started out as a simple mixture of natural ingredients: beef tallow and milk. We can thank France for this. Napoleon III sought to make poor people happier by giving them access to an inexpensive butter substitute. The industrious Emperor held a contest and the winner was French chemist Hippolyte Mège-Mouriès. In 1869, Mège-Mouriès created a process for churning beef tallow with milk and called it oleo-margarine, thereby winning the Emperor's prize.

The French didn't like oleo-margarine, presumably due to the white-grey color. But Mège-Mouriès sold the patent to the Dutch who dyed it buttery yellow. Yellow fake butter was acceptable, and eventually the company making the yellow margarine was bought by Unilever, which makes soaps by a related process.

Margarine was initially resisted by the food industry, ironically the same industry that would decades later force it into every processed food product and restaurant in the nation. The political force at the time were dairy farmers who lobbied their wallets and slowed margarine's market primarily by banning the yellow dye and forcing companies to dye margarine pink instead.

Margarine sales did increase during World War II. When wartime butter scarcity forced consumers to switch to margarine, consumers realized that it tasted fine and that the pink color made little difference in baked goods. In 1950, the U.S. government repealed the heavy margarine tax, and the market continued to grow as individual states reversed their bans on yellow-colored margarine. The last state to repeal the dye ban was Wisconsin which not coincidentally had less heart disease in later decades despite being one of the more obese states in the nation.

With margarine bans gone, food manufacturers turned their money toward health policy politics, starting by assuaging the American Heart Association's early attempts to discourage margarine use, then by incorporating their product into dietary guidelines and nutritional counseling. Currently related food industry advertising promises unfounded health benefits.

Given the intended audience, let's look at some numbers without getting into statistical games.

So just how much margarine did we eat? A lot. Margarine consumption doubled to over 10 pounds per person per year after World War II. In fact, following World War II margarine increasingly replaced butter for fifty years and we still haven't reached the low numbers of 1909 where margarine use was rare and so was heart disease. Margarine use surpassed butter in the 1950s and continues to lead consumption. The graph trend below shows the alarming history of butter replacement by margarine in our diets.

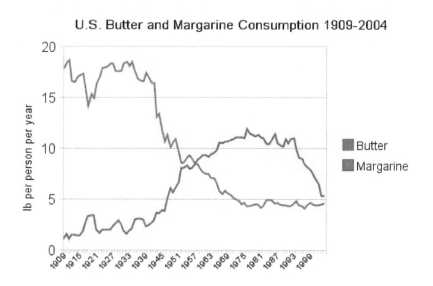

U.S. Butter and Margarine Consumption 1909-2004

Heart disease resulting in loss of blood flow to the heart (heart attack) was first described in 1912 by Dr. James B. Herrick.   Heart disease was considered rare in the 19th century and remains rare in many countries today. This could not have resulted from gross under diagnosis because major heart attacks have characteristic symptoms, such as chest pain/pressure that usually includes arm, jaw or neck and severe heart attacks have measurable changes in blood flow parameters. Physicians up to that time were regularly diagnosing other heart conditions, such as infections or arrhythmias, so heart attacks would hardly have been missed.

The following graph is of total heart disease deaths in the United States from 1900 to 2005. It represents all types of heart disease deaths, including congestive heart failure, arrhythmia and myocarditis (a heart infection usually caused by a virus).

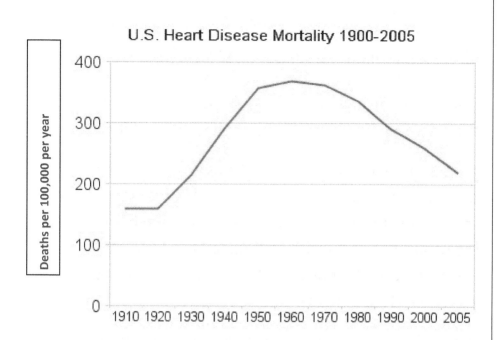

U.S. Heart Disease Mortality 1900-2005

Keeping in mind that while death (mortality) from heart disease has been falling since the 1950s due to improved medical treatment, numbers of people getting heart disease has not. Physicians are simply much better at keeping people alive in the 21st century, but we haven't stopped heart disease because we haven't stopped eating fake fats and oils. Despite all the advances in medicine, our death rate from heart disease is *higher* now than it was over a century ago.

These are not subtle numbers. Imagine the political power needed to keep this quiet for fifty years. Another negative health outcome was that, as arteries clogged slowly more people developed heart rhythm problems, commonly known as atrial fibrillation ("a-fib"). To keep a-fib hearts from clotting, we give patients Coumadin. Coumadin inhibits vitamin K. Vitamin K is important in stopping atherosclerosis (hardening of the arteries). And what is a common source of vitamin K? Yes — butter.

In one action, U.S. health policy removed from our diet a substance that kept us from forming plaque in our arteries *and* promoted an artificial substance that by itself accelerated artery blockage. Remember, these data trends were evident nearly 50 years ago, and we are still eating nearly as much fake fat as butter.

Decreasing butter consumption and increasing *trans* fat consumption contributed to the massive incidence of CHD (chronic heart disease) seen in the United States and other industrial nations today. Remember France — that country that rejected margarine and kept on eating butter? France has the highest per-capita dairy fat consumption of any industrial nation, along with a comparatively low intake of hydrogenated fat, *but* has the second-lowest rate of CHD, just behind Japan.

Heart disease was rare in developed nations at the turn of the century. Between 1920 and 1960, the incidence of heart disease rose, becoming the nation's number one killer. During the same period, butter consumption plummeted from eighteen pounds per person per year to four while margarine consumption both directly and through processed foods, skyrocketed. By itself this is not proof, but it should have been sufficient to pause both the medical community and the health policy agencies. Eventually, the medical community responded but now battled an entrenched false concept in the general public that butter was bad and margarine was good.

Margarine's nemesis has been Harvard University's Medical School. In 1994, Harvard University researchers reported that people who ate partially hydrogenated oils, which are high in trans fats, had nearly twice the risk of heart attacks as those who consumed much less trans fats. In an analysis of the Framingham study, Harvard researchers proved that harmful effects of margarine increases over time — harm measurable more than a decade after consumption.[50] Several other large studies in the United States, including the Nurses' Health Study conducted by researchers at the Harvard School of Public Health, have demonstrated a strong link between earlier death and consumption of foods high in trans fat.

Meanwhile, Harvard had a wily foe in the food industry. While food industry money delayed public focus on trans

---

[50] Margarine intake and subsequent coronary heart disease in men. Gillman MW1, Cupples LA, Gagnon D, et al. Epidemiology. 1997 Mar;8(2):144-9.

fats, food chemists modified their laboratory manufacturing to continue producing artificial compounds that are not classified as "trans" yet have an architecture completely unnatural to the body.

Eventually the trans-fat message made it to the public. When the public outcry became great enough, not even political contributions could stop the anti-trans-fat movement, starting with New York City's notoriously reactive ban. Even this, however, was a misrepresentation of the data.

Recall our cis and trans fat discussion from the prior chapter on fats.

Some trans fats occur naturally in small amounts in some foods, including meat and dairy products, but most trans fats in the American diet are formed when vegetable oils are chemically changed to give them a longer shelf life. Cookies, potato chips, baked products, and similar manufactured foods are particularly loaded with trans fats. A narrow-minded conclusion to this might be to substitute all saturated fats with unsaturated fats. However, there is evidence that changing the natural balance of saturated fats to unsaturated fats could also cause harm, demonstrating again that premature marketing of substances such as plant sterols[51] to

_____

[51] Plant sterols are plant compounds similar in structure to cholesterol.

decrease heart disease[52] could have the opposite effect and cause harm[53]. Naturally-occurring trans fats in naturally-occurring foods as part of a balanced diet may be safe. We simply do not know.

Nevertheless, the federal government passed regulations requiring that by 2006 all food labels disclose how much trans fat a product contains, swinging the pendulum in the opposite direction by leaping at the behest of political pressure[54]. The government could have said "avoid processed foods." This would be an appropriate warning avoiding the error now occurring as artificial (hydrogenated) oils are being packaged as "no trans fats", tricking consumers into believing this is a healthful choice. There is *no evidence* that chemically transformed fats and oils are safe for consumption — whether or not the product contains trans fats.

And the data? Remember the data history before margarine showing hardly any heart disease from natural

---

[52] Association of plasma noncholesterol sterol levels with severity of coronary heart disease. Sutherland W, Williams M, Nye E. Nutr Metab Cardiovasc Dis 1998;8:386-391

[53] Controversial role of plant sterol esters in the management of hypercholesterolaemia. Weingärtner O; Böhm M; Laufs U. DOI: http://dx.doi.org/10.1093/eurheartj/ehn580404-409. 2009

[54]

http://www.snopes.com/food/warnings/butter.asp#lxtH3IollWWLOjiG.99

fats. The bottom line has been the same in all the research: Natural oils, such as olive oil and canola oil, are preferable to any hydrogenated fat, either solid or semisolid. The evidence has been there all along. The 1940's and 50's did not show that margarine is better than butter but rather that unsaturated fat is better than saturated fat. A message of "eat less beef" was opposed by cattle farmers so it was never heard. A message of "avoid artificial oils such as margarine" never had a chance politically. Even the American Heart Association was silenced from the proposed "avoid trans fats and hydrogenated oils" and directed to only say "avoid heavily hydrogenated oils" such as stick margarine.

This was in the 1960s. Twenty years later physicians (and everyone else) were still pushing margarine on patients as a method of lowering cholesterol and, ironically, heart attack and stroke risk. To our discredit, healthcare providers have encouraged use of margarine without appropriate data. To the shame of my profession, in the 1980s I remember we specifically told post-heart attack patients in Detroit and Chicago to eat margarine and never use butter. To assist, the dieticians ensured that margarine was on every hospital tray in the cardiac care unit.

This is the power of food manufacturers on our politicians and medical organizations. In short, government guidelines are not based upon well-rounded science. Government guidelines are based upon who has the most political clout. For detailed information on these unfortunate events in health policy or if you simply wish to be further incensed about how the U.S. government negatively influenced your health, I recommend reading Gyorgy Scrinis' text *Nutritionism: The Science and Politics of Dietary Advice.*

Food Pyramid Problems

Beginning in 1943 the United States, through the USDA and National Academy of Science, published an unscientific food wheel giving equal weight in the diet to 7 food categories; vegetables, fruit, bread, butter, dairy, meat and potato/starch. The political climate in the 1940s, despite World War II, was clearly pro-butter. This climate would shift completely within three decades.

Even in the 1940s, science was advanced sufficiently to have stopped inaccurate redundancies, but it did not. There was no basis for the recommendation and it remains a major nutritional folly by the United States in nutritional manipulation. To their credit, the food wheel sought to recommend a variety of foods and did not endorse artificial substances. This would also shift within three decades.

The food wheel would soon be replaced by increasingly misleading guidance.

By 1956, the government indoctrinated school children and the general public with a "4 squares" guideline. This set the stage for alarmingly increasing cancer rates we see today: equal weight to dairy, meat, vegetable/fruit and bread. It also led to the looks of utter disbelief when patients in my rural clinic hear that they do not need to eat meat at all to be healthy, much less with every meal.

Two decades later, the 1970s repeated the same mistake of four basic food groups. While some would begin heeding the advice of moderation in all groups, the broad view by the public resulted in no change in eating behavior, sending yet another generation to the oncologists and cardiac surgeons while setting the groundwork for the obesity/diabetes epidemic. By then, food manufacturing held tremendous political clout which turned mediocre advice into, at best, useless fodder. The unhealthy practices that food manufacturers used was brought to public light in *Food for Nought* in 1974; the backlash served to increase the lobbying efforts to protect against decline of support and to decrease the quality of food further.

Medical science knew in the 1970s which general eating habits were associated with serious chronic illness. By the 1970s, medicine would have advocated "eat less meat" were it not for the food industry politicking which turned the message into "eat less saturated fat," a meaningless term to the general public at the time.

Indeed, the medical community was increasingly skeptical. The 1970s produced several nutritionally-impactful books touching both directly and tangentially on how the food industrial complex caused health problems — *The Saccharin Disease, Fabricated Foods, Pounds and Inches* and *Dr Atkins Diet Revolution*. It isn't that we didn't know better. The health policy agencies and the academic institutions financially controlled by government health policy agencies belittled those books' attempts to warn the public.

These published educated skeptics were mentioned but largely ignored at major medical institutions in the 1980s and early 1990s. Any book or publication, academic or otherwise, can be severely critiqued. Ripping someone else's opinions apart is intellectually fun and can even be collegial at times, but the responsible intellect always seriously asks "*what can we learn from this*." Why the public health sector did not allow this question to be asked I leave to the reader's ponderings.

By 1992 an actual food "pyramid" appeared. The strong base of cereal grains and breads accelerated the obesity/diabetes epidemic ensuring that type 2 diabetes mellitus would worsen to encompass even children.

Animal protein from meats and dairy still comprised a 1:1 ratio with vegetables and fruits despite conclusive irrefutable findings that plant-based diets reduced major chronic disease. While the recommendations for fats and oils were reduced, no distinction was made between "good" fats and "bad" fats. Additionally, animal products were not promoted as fats, thereby ensuring that Americans following government guidelines consumed at least three times more fats, mostly concentrated saturated or hydrogenated, than would be healthy in a nutritionally balanced diet.

By 2003, the food pyramid morphed only from a cartoon perspective and the misinformation from 1992 progressed yet another decade. By 2011, this was addressed to suggest that half of our foods should be fruit and vegetables, leaving far too many grains on our plates and more than twice the protein needed for optimal health.

In the end, over 70 years of government misdirection on nutrition continues to run contrary to healthy biochemical metabolism. How U.S. health policy allowed the food industry this insult to our health may be explored in the previously cited textbook *Nutritionism : The Science and Politics of Dietary Advice*.

All of the misinformation could have been averted by remaining silent. However, a beneficent government would inform consumers that the less meat they eat, the healthier they will be. Further advice should have stated that processed and refined foods, including most grain products, should not be consumed regularly[55].

Although there was solid mortality data on the risks of being overweight, food guidelines did not inform people to eat less but instead encouraged overeating. There was no data suggesting the government recommendations were valid in a healthful way. The ongoing recommendations then and now served political rather than health-oriented outcomes. Government health policy is primarily a justification for the budget of policy agencies. The result is always harm by ignorance.

"Unless we put medical freedom into the constitution, the time will come when medicine will organize itself into an undercover dictatorship . . . denying equal privileges. All such laws are un-American and despotic . . . "

—Benjamin Rush, Physician, Signer of Declaration of Independence

---

[55] Hall RH. The Unofficial Guide to Smart Nutrition. 2000. IDG Books Worldwide. Foster City CA.

Don't spoil a good (fermented) thing

"I have wished to see chemistry applied to domestic objects, to malting, for instance, brewing, making cider, to fermentation and distillation generally, to the making of bread, butter, cheese, soap, to the incubation of eggs"
—Thomas Jefferson

"There's just a little mold on top, it's fine."
—Renate Hetzner

As discussed in earlier chapters, our body is designed to live symbiotically with nature. Ancient people without that ability died out and did not pass their traits on to us. This commonsense approach, a part of everyday life for millennia, is somehow being reinvented by markets rebranding a "microbiome" for capitalistic purposes. If coining new terms for ancient concepts helps people choose a healthier diet, on the other hand, why not? While the term "microbiome" may help some persons understand why they should be cautious using supplements and pharmaceuticals that easily disrupt the natural microbe balance, supporting our gut microbiome predates civilization.

The microbiome isn't new. The microbiome is ancient, completely natural and doesn't come in a pill. That won't stop people, even physician authors, from marketing supplements and scaring you into buying their commercial brand, but somewhere along the line, more real food may find its way into the American diet.

The concept of fermenting food by keeping it edible and nutritious for our body for long periods of time without either refrigeration or industrial food manufacturing was well-practiced by humans until the industrial age made sterilized food convenient and inexpensive. Using ancient methods properly is safe; the fact that we exist to read this is the evidence. Persons using ancient knowledge today are considered quaint or faddish, however preserving food with simple fermentation or dehydration makes sense and does not require any external power source to process and maintain the food.

The safe food preservation method is placing food in an environment that is unfriendly or deadly to microorganisms that are unfriendly or deadly to our bodies.

Food preserved in a way that sucks all the water out of any bacteria unfortunate enough to land on the food cannot spoil easily. Dried or dehydrated foods keep well at room temperature in this way. Another way to achieve food preservation is through liquids that dehydrate — brine and sugars. In ancient times, salt and honey would be used.

The food method most interesting today, however, is fermentation. Fermentation is simply a controlled rot with microorganisms that will not harm us but which so predominate in the food that harmful bacteria (and fungus) cannot compete.

The fermentation can either directly or indirectly prevent contamination by deadly bacteria. If the good fermenter, such as Saccharomyces Cerevisae (yeast) produces a lot of waste product, such as alcohol, the harmful bacteria cannot grow in the fluid. The fluid is safe within reason to drink, often for years. If the good fermenter is another bacteria, it will compete with or kill off harmful bacteria and outnumber the harmful bacteria so badly that the bad bacteria cannot reproduce. The most common are the lactobacilli — the fermenters that give us yogurt and kefir. Some cultures yield cheese. Similar processes occur for fermented vegetables, most commonly from the cabbage family but other vegetables can be fermented as well. Leuconostoc mesenteroides is one helpful bacteria found in barrel-aged sauerkraut.

Aspergillus oryzae, a fungus, is the friendly fermenter for miso — a mixture of soybeans and various types of grain. Soybeans can also be fermented with *Rhizopus oryzae* or *Rhizopus oligosporus,* two other friendly fungi, but the result is then tempeh, with a different flavor and texture than miso.

Many fermented foods and beverages have more than one healthful fermenter, and may have a combination of both beneficial bacteria and friendly fungi, such as Kombucha tea (which is a fermented tea, not a "mushroom" tea despite that the colony at the top of the culture resembles a mushroom).

The microbiology specifics help to demonstrate that including fermented foods in the diet is beneficial to the body, not harmful. The post-antibiotic era erroneously taught us all germs are bad. In fact, many germs are not only harmless but can also improve and sustain our health. Now science is increasingly demonstrating that microbes in our bodies are helpful and probably necessary for proper health.

Microbes produce nutrients that our body requires for normal function. For example, vitamin B12 (cyanocobalamin) is necessary for life but is only made by bacteria. To make this compound, the bacteria require the trace element cobalt. Cobalt is found in tiny amounts in the soil; cobalt can be easily depleted from the soil. Here is another example: Certain compounds in soy can only be broken down by fungus enzymes found in miso, which additionally contains some unique antioxidants. Thus this fungus actually makes soy-based food more nutritious to humans.

Health providers are erroneously taught in medical school that the only way to meet the B12 requirement of the body is by ingesting animal products, such as meat and eggs, or by taking a supplement. This is wrong. History teaches us that this is wrong, yet even at my contrarian best I did not question this during training — nor did any of my vegan classmates from India.

There are peoples that go through their entire lives eating only plants. You can find many of them in India where they do not suffer from vitamin B12 deficiency. This natural example should have caused medical scientists to suspect that B12 is not made by animals. The Indians are getting B12 from their guts because by eating a vegan diet *and* not taking antibiotics they have fostered symbiotic bacteria in their gut that make B12.

The entire human gut is over 30 feet long and filled from lips to anus with microorganisms in addition to the enzymes and secretions made by the gut lining itself. The number of microorganisms in the healthy human gut far exceeds the number of human cells. What most persons call digestion is essentially fermentation done rapidly — the human body cannot wait several weeks for the food we consume to turn into energy. In the human body, we achieve this quick rotting of food by modifying the pH and the enzyme content of the food throughout the course of the gut.

Enzymes needed to digest simple sugars are present in saliva and can be absorbed within minutes. In the normal stomach, the acid level is very high (which means the pH is very low), further decomposing the food while killing many microorganisms that get swallowed — such as virus particles and certain bacteria. Stomach enzymes, two of which are pepsin and rennin, begin breaking down the food so that the next set of enzymes from the pancreas, trypsin and lipase, can complete the process in a low acid ("basic" or high pH) section of gut called the small intestine. The fermentation largely completes as food travels through the small intestine where additional enzymes can squeeze the last bit of energy and nutrients from the food before entering the large intestine which absorbs water prior to bowel movement leading to the excretion of waste we call stool.

This process takes about 24 hours — much faster than fermentation left to some microorganisms in a crock. Due to the length of the human gut and several muscular valves between sections, the body can digest meals in rapid succession and keep the stomach contents in the stomach until ready to proceed to the small intestine. The gut even informs the downstream tissues that food is coming. We call this peristalsis; that information usually creates some urge to defecate within 30 minutes of eating.

The point of the anatomy review is to demonstrate that fermentation is not something to fear. Humans ferment food within our own bodies on a grand scale and call it digestion.

While the fortunate grew up with grandparents (or parents) who still used fermentation methods to preserve the harvest, most persons in industrialized nations were not so fortunate. These unfortunate persons will be understandably skeptical. For those wary, starting with packaged products that say "contains live cultures", such as yoghurt, kefir and miso may be a comfortable start. (Don't cook the *live cultures* or they become *dead* cultures.) From there, branch out to fermented vegetables like sauerkraut, tempeh and kimchee.

Pick up some organic apple cider (fermented apples). Sprinkle some organic apple cider vinegar on your salad and be amazed that you did not get sick from fungus.

After acclimating and learning the taste of these and experiencing that the "germs" didn't even make you ill, explore your local health food store to purchase fermented vegetable products that are not pasteurized. These will be refrigerated, although most needn't be. Visit a local farm or Amish community that produces these products and learn to make your own fermented vegetables in a crock (or large glass jar) at home.

Although not this book's focus, your skin also contains helpful microogranisms (and even small insects) that do not harm you and can reduce your exposure and risk from other less friendly threats.

In summary, many microorganisms can live in and on your body without causing any harm. Science continues discerning why those microorganisms need to be part of the body to maintain good health. There is no need to fear the organisms that have lived symbiotically within humans for millennia — we have imbalanced our health and our lives in erroneous attempts to be germ-free.

Not doing anything different IS the problem

"Insanity is doing the same thing over and over again and expecting different results."
—Albert Einstein
"I'm beautiful in my way
'Cause God makes no mistakes
I'm on the right track, baby I was born this way."
—Lady Gaga

"You weren't born obese. God didn't do that."
—Dr Frank

This was the most difficult chapter to write: informing readers that the reason they are sick, fat and tired is simply because of one's own choices. Every day we make choices that will determine if we move our body toward health or toward illness. We have discussed how food choices can hurt us. The key understanding of patients who lost weight and kept it off is this: There is no quick easy fat fix; it is a lifelong commitment. But patients also tell me this: the key understanding is only acceptable once they understand how the body works.

Thus, this discussion would be incomplete without the topics of how we eat and why we eat. Failing to understand one's motive for poor food choices translates to a failure to stay thin. The desired outcome is to eat the right amount of natural foods because our body needs it — not for any other reason.

The Right amount of Balanced Foods

The denial mechanism for most persons is rationalizing their behavior by comparing themselves with someone who makes similar choices or with someone who appears to be an exception to the rules of health. "At least I'm not as unhealthy as _____" will never solve your problem. Being content with poor dietary choices because your shopping cart contains fewer processed foods than someone at Walmart who is so obese they must use an electric scooter cart will never improve your own health.

Bad choices don't make deals with you; bad choices are simply bad choices.

Smoking less than someone else or drinking less than someone else does absolutely nothing to protect your health. I have not in nearly three decades of practice found a 70 year-old who smoked in moderation or was obese but was still healthy. Conversely, I have many 70 year-olds in my practice who did not smoke or drink who still work full-time, exercise regularly and are much healthier physically, indeed look better physically, than the fat forty year-olds who drink and smoke in moderation.

Once I had a 42 year-old patient who was facing death due to his poor choices. His heart would no longer pump adequately to his obese body. His arteries were too clogged to bypass and he was therefore on a heart transplant list. Because I've had patients die waiting for a replacement heart I am extremely strict with these patients. In addition to traditional medical regimens, I put him on a vegan diet — one of the only things left that might save him.[56] The patient didn't complain. But his mother, she who taught him the horrid food habits, criticized me (in front of the patient no less) for "fat-shaming" him.

I do not suffer from an excess of tact, even less so when a patient's life is on the line. So I lectured to her that had she fat-shamed him thirty years ago he wouldn't be dying. Sometimes the truth hurts. Yes I needed the bully-pulpit of a physician to back her down and as a result her son is still alive today. I don't care whether she thinks I am nice or not, I care that her son still has a chance at life.

Being fat doesn't mean you're a bad person only that it is bad for your health. The mother might not have known margarine was bad, but no one has ever suggested morbid obesity and diabetes are healthy. She made bad choices and so did her son, until he learned otherwise. Enabling a loved one's obesity with unhealthy food is no different than giving an alcoholic family member alcohol.

---

[56] Forks over Knives. Ibid.

Thus I am shamelessly "fat-shaming", fake food-shaming, tobacco-shaming, alcohol-shaming and sloth-shaming my patients into better health. While more specifics of healthier living are in the last chapter, the rationale and strategy are in this chapter. Each decision made about food is an opportunity for health.

Earlier we explored how fat tissue makes us unhealthy in many ways. Animals were not designed to stay fat. Belly fat exists simply to get animals through months of lean times — frozen months or drought — which humans and other domestic animals no longer face. While *what* we eat is most important, *how much* and *why* we eat is the next concern.

Let us dispel the myth that a person can be fat and healthy. Were that the case, the number of fat people would be reasonably constant in history and normal people would die sooner. Alternatively, as obesity increased, health would also increase. This is not the case.

What is the history of obesity in the United States? Let's graph it.

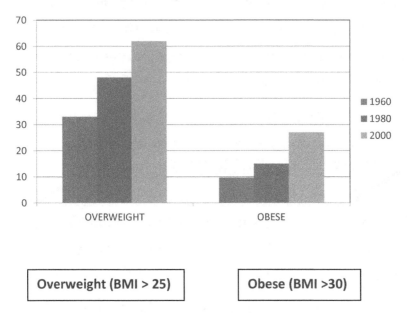

Percentage Overweight & Obesity the in United States

	1960
	1980
	2000

OVERWEIGHT   OBESE

| Overweight (BMI > 25) | Obese (BMI >30) |

In the U.S., persons overweight nearly DOUBLED from 1960 to 2000 and the number of obese nearly tripled. Diabetes rates rose from 0.9% to 7% in that same time frame — an increase of 7 times[57]. Already established as a cause of diabetes, something in addition to fat is causing our bodies to fall out of balance. Now that you've read most of this book, you can probably guess what else is poisoning us.

---

[57] CDC's Division of Diabetes Translation. National Diabetes Surveillance System available at http://www.cdc.gov/diabetes/statistics

Fat also causes cancer. The incidence of new cancer cases increases each year in the United States,[58] the only notable exception being the temporary decrease in colon cancer cases as a result of physicians removing precancerous tissue (polyps) during recommended colonoscopy screening.

To be healthy, the human body needs a balance of the right foods in the right amounts. If you are not eating the right foods in the right amounts, you are or will soon be fat, sick or tired. Because America is getting fatter and sicker, the path most Americans take is evident. There is no shortcut to the solution of healthy eating and there is no end to this solution. While there is no alternative to this solution, it is an *easy* solution. Our ancestors managed it with no education and only living off the land. Only eat completely whole natural foods grown in a completely natural environment.

There is no more "is this on my diet?" If it is made by man, spit it out. If it has a label, you should be extremely cautious. If it has a label with anything you do not recognize as a plant or animal, do not eat it or drink it. If that is too much work, then go simpler still: if you wouldn't recognize it on a farm, in a forest or swimming in a lake, don't eat it or drink it. (The organic versus

---

[58]

http://seer.cancer.gov/archive/csr/1975_2001/results_merged/topic_delay.pdf

conventional discussion has been covered and will not be repeated here.)

What is the correct amount of food? The amount that causes your body to return to a normal size. Your body fat content can be estimated from internet charts on Body Mass Index unless you are pregnant or a competitive body builder, in which case your health care provider can do a more detailed fat analysis. There are some problems with BMI charts as they look at a normal population at a particular age, but it is a reasonable starting point.

How do I know you're overweight? Well for one, you're reading a book about it. But that aside, let's look at the numbers. These numbers essentially link your fat level to risk of death. This death risk is real and measurable. The insurance companies use this to charge you more for life insurance the fatter you are — these are real numbers with real impact.

For example, if you are 6 feet tall and weigh more than 180 pounds, you are overweight and will die sooner (all things being equal) than you would at 160 pounds or even 140 pounds. In general, you add roughly 5 pounds of healthy weight per inch. 5 feet tall? Your maximum weight should be about 120. Even if you are 6' 4" you shouldn't weigh over 200 pounds. If you are shocked by these facts, I am glad you are reading this book.

However, your total body weight is just the *start*. You can still fail the fat test if your body weight is normal *and* you carry fat around your waist. Thus, even the self-proclaimed athletes can be obese as the waistline restriction still applies to all but pregnant patients. This should disabuse those who in their own mind are athletes but justifying their obesity by time spent in the gym. If your waist is more than 34 inches (male) or 32 inches (female), you are probably not an athlete and you are most probably fat. Let's explore this more using your own body as an example.

To achieve this, refer to the BMI chart on the next page. To determine your BMI, find your height on the leftmost column, follow it across the row until you reach your closest body weight. From there trace directly up to the top row to find your BMI. In this chart, if you are not in the white section, you are unquestionably fat. If you are completely above the chart, that is the realm of the morbidly obese and you need to take urgent action.

Adult BMI Chart

BMI Height	19	20	21	22	23	24	25	26	27	28	29	30	31	32	33	34	35
							Weight in Pounds										
4'10"	91	96	100	105	110	115	119	124	129	134	138	143	148	153	158	162	167
4'11"	94	99	104	109	114	119	124	128	133	138	143	148	153	158	163	168	173
5'	97	102	107	112	118	123	128	133	138	143	148	153	158	163	168	174	179
5'1"	100	106	111	116	122	127	132	137	143	148	153	158	164	169	174	180	185
5'2"	104	109	115	120	126	131	136	142	147	153	158	164	169	175	180	186	191
5'3"	107	113	118	124	130	135	141	146	152	158	163	169	175	180	186	191	197
5'4"	110	116	122	128	134	140	145	151	157	163	169	174	180	186	192	197	204
5'5"	114	120	123	132	138	144	150	156	162	168	174	180	186	192	198	204	210
5'6"	118	124	130	136	142	148	155	161	167	173	179	186	192	198	204	210	216
5'7"	121	127	134	140	146	153	159	166	172	178	185	191	198	204	211	217	223
5'8"	125	131	138	144	151	158	164	171	177	184	190	197	203	210	216	223	230
5'9"	128	135	142	149	155	162	169	176	182	189	196	203	209	216	223	230	236
5'10"	132	139	146	153	160	167	174	181	188	195	202	209	216	222	229	236	243
5'11"	136	143	150	157	165	172	179	186	193	200	208	215	222	229	236	243	250
6'	140	147	154	162	169	177	184	191	199	206	213	221	228	235	242	250	258
6'1"	144	151	159	166	174	182	189	197	204	212	219	227	235	242	250	257	265
6'2"	148	155	163	171	179	186	194	202	210	218	225	233	241	249	256	264	272
6'3"	152	160	168	176	184	192	200	208	216	224	232	240	248	256	264	272	279
	Healthy Weight						Overweight					Obese					

Most people should not need a BMI chart. Assuming average heights, men with waists over 34 inches are overweight; women with waists over 32 inches are overweight. If you were in excellent physical shape when you graduated from high school, that is the weight you should never exceed. Once your spine begins to shrink — usually noticeable by our fifth decade — you should weigh even less. It is a common misconception that we should gain weight as we age. To be healthy we should *lose* weight as we age, unless we are gaining pure muscle or are pregnant (the latter being temporary weight gain).

The old adage "You can never be too rich or too thin" is true. As it turns out, you cannot be too thin — unless of course you have an eating disorder. But there is no research showing any benefit for being fat. You can in fact have a normal BMI and still be in poor health from obesity-related conditions simply by having too much belly fat.

The waist size must actually be measured. Using waist size listed on your pants will not work because fat people wear their pants below their true waist. However, there is a useful test using pants size: if the inseam number is lower than the waist number, you are overweight.

Further, there are some newer developments showing that you live longer the thinner you are and longevity is best realized at 20% lower than "normal"; normal being weight in the non-shaded area of the BMI chart. The data confuses some people who read that thin elderly people die earlier than overweight elderly people. Why? Because elderly people who were normal or fat *and then* lost weight unintentionally did so because they are dying of *something else*. Their low weight was the result of their disease, not the cause of their disease. Any disease that burns a lot of calories, such as emphysema (COPD), cancer and chronic infections, can cause patients to lose weight, often over a few years, before they die. They don't die because they are thin; they die because they are sick and lost weight trying to fight the sickness.

Pertinent to this topic is weight loss speed. It is not healthy to drive significant weight loss for months. When my patients choose to return to normal weight, limiting rapid weight loss to 40 days usually yields about twenty pounds of actual fat loss - it takes a bit less than a pound of fat a day to run the body and the necessary components for fat mobilization require certain macronutrients to stop the body from breaking down muscle for energy.

Although laboratory calculations equate one pound of fat to equal 3500 calories, in clinical practice that doesn't appear to hold up. It clearly cannot account for my patients who document 1200 or fewer calories a day, exercise daily and still gain fat weight while academic authorities tell us it takes at least 2000 calories a day to run the body. That is why I rarely ask patients to count calories; it doesn't work well. Nor does any of the reductionist thinking that drives the supplement industry we discussed in earlier chapters.

When I myself have measured calories at 2000 I gain fat weight unless I burn at least 300 calories doing physical exercise. Exercising at 300 calories a day is not an "average" adult activity in America unfortunately. If I eat 1600 calories I maintain my weight, which is 162 pounds on a 71 inch tall, 31 inch waist frame. So I'm taller than average, thinner than average and more athletic than average but I burn at least 20% *fewer* calories than the average person is supposed to?

We have been conditioned to eat a daily amount that results in obesity. We have also been duped into thinking that what works in a laboratory test tube will work in our bodies the same way it did in the lab. We are told to think this despite thousands of variables in our body that the laboratory cannot account for or duplicate.

I can put similarly-sized patients on approximately 500 calorie monitored diet (I tell them what and how much to eat not how many calories to eat) and one will lose nearly a pound daily while the other will lose a pound every three days. Medical science simply does not adequately understand nutrition to be issuing ultimatums as true for all patients. For this reason, rapid weight loss should be monitored closely by a physician and not by a math program on your Fit Bit. Your needs are not average and your needs will change over time.

Rapid weight loss should be supervised by a physician and likely includes blood tests and, for patients with other medical illnesses, monitoring medications. Patients I supervise reduce their medications by at least thirty percent within a month. *Unsupervised* rapid weight loss would have left those patients overmedicated and, as a result, perhaps dead. This is a reason you should *never* tell a friend to try your weight loss program by mimicking what you have done.

Consuming fewer calories should drop your metabolism. Your blood pressure will drop. Your blood sugar will drop. Your sleep will improve. Losing fat properly should feel *good* not like a struggle.

After the rapid weight loss, which represents a natural state of relative starvation experienced by our ancestors, a gradual increase in specific healthy foods should occur to either maintain the goal weight or reduce the fat loss rate. There is always an initial weight gain with any increase in natural food: there is more substance in the gastrointestinal tract to weigh and there is more water held within that same food. This is not *fat* gain, it is weight gain and there is a difference. This can be the time to introduce specific exercise to restore any lost muscle, drive growth hormone production and increase the metabolic rates.

Too much of a good thing isn't good

Fake foods aside, we eat too much.

Why? When asked, most people can tell you why they eat — hunger, reward, boredom and habit are major reasons.

Hunger is a signal that your body can consume more food. It is normal to feel hungry. You should feel hungry most all the time, just as our ancestors did. Hunger is completely useless in industrial countries and learning to acknowledge and then ignore hunger is necessary to maintaining healthy weight.

 Acknowledge hunger, do not satisfy hunger. You *should* feel hungry most of the time, just like you should feel the need to breath most of the time. Again, hunger has been marketed to make you believe it is evil and should be eradicated. Quite the opposite — hunger should be encouraged and malnutrition should be eradicated. Never believe that we have a hunger problem in North America — we have an obesity problem from too much food and too poor food quality.

Feeling hungry is normal.

Feeling hungry is normal .

Feeling hungry is normal .

Often what adults interpret as hunger is thirst. Drinking more water reduces the sensation of hunger and also causes people to eat less food even though no energy was consumed by drinking water. Persons who routinely drink a glass of water before meals or consume broth-based soup before meals eat fewer calories and report no more hunger when compared to those persons who do not. If it were hunger or true energy need rather than thirst driving them, there would be no difference in calorie consumption.

Our food choices also influence the hunger sensation. Persons eating simple carbohydrates such as breads, pasta and rice will feel hungry much earlier and often more intensely than will persons eating natural foods. Those who have protein with their meals report feeling satisfied for more hours than those who have low protein meals.

Some persons use food as a reward; the extreme of this is a complex mental disorder called bulemia. Rewarding oneself with food is one way to ensure you will not maintain a healthy weight, even intermittent rewards are recipes for weight gain. Food rewards exchanged for exercising an extra hour or not eating all day teaches you disappointment when you do not obtain the reward food.

Further, the food rewards are rarely healthy. In 30 years I have never heard a patient say "I ran twenty extra minutes so when I get home I'm going to have a carrot!" The reward food usually over-replaces the calories burned or skipped. Does that mean you can never have ice cream or chocolate again? No, it means you plan for it to be part of your food that day, and you eat a very small portion that you can control. For a restaurant meal, start by splitting a small dessert with everyone at the table; most of the pleasure in desserts are from the first bite.

Boredom is another reason people overeat. Boredom is closely-linked to habit but there are some differences. Bored eaters tend to eat when they are not doing anything exciting or entertaining. Watching a boring television show or waiting for the laundry to complete, sitting at an athletic event when your child isn't playing, attending a meeting or conference with dull speakers, waiting for your family to get home for dinner... there are as many boring things in life as there are poor food choices. Food helps pass the time while rewarding your patience. Boredom is an easy fix. Replacing the snacking with water, tea or chewing gum are healthy switches. And finding something else to do, such as a crossword puzzle, cleaning the garage, walking the dog or calling a friend can also break up the monotony.

Habit is harder to overcome because breaking a habit is emotionally painful. We are animals and animals prefer routine, as any pet owner will tell you. You have had decades longer than your dog to ingrain your habitual behavior, yet it takes a lot of patience to break a dog of a habit, whether the habit be bad or neutral. Worse, your habits can also have a positive impact — take the common habit of family evening dinner as an example.

Family dinner was once a habit for most everyone. While this is no longer commonplace, there are social benefits to families, particularly families with children, to regularly scheduled family dinner. The structure and time is habitual. The expectation is frequently large comfort meals, so keeping the structure and time while modifying the food types is possible. Remain mindful that this type of change is harder for children than for adults. Gradual changes work better with children, starting with smaller and smarter entrees and fruit or sweetened tea for dessert. The first change in our family dinner was to stop serving bread or rolls at meals.

Eating lunch at noon is a habit. We don't need to eat three meals a day, it is simply a habit. Taking an hour to eat lunch is a habit. Going to a restaurant or ordering out for food is a habit. Each food decision moves you toward or away from health. If lunch cannot be skipped, try replacing the larger meal in the cafeteria with an apple, a bottle of water and a walk outside. Order one entrée and split it with a coworker. Turn each habit into a decision.

Your personal environment is full of decisions. The decision might be choosing between a packaged meal or a piece of fresh fruit. The decision might be to simply not purchase a chemical you would otherwise spray around your house. It could be adding organic cream or soymilk to your coffee rather than the chemical bomb of flavors made in a laboratory. It might mean having your organic coffee or tea black when you have no healthy options or flavoring it with a dash of herbs like cinnamon or stevia.

There are other decisions requiring more commitment. One example is deciding to go to yoga several times a week instead of relying on a pain pill that harms your kidneys, raises your blood pressure and increases your blood clot risk. Another example could be deciding to save the usual dinner plates for Thanksgiving only and use your dessert plates as a size gauge for a meal. (Inherent in that decision is not eating second helpings.)

Each healthy decision you make will help detoxify your body. Fat is an inflammatory tissue. Fat makes you feel sick and tired, perhaps because when you feel sick and tired you are more likely to restrict your movement and sleep more. Feeling sick and tired is nature's perfect way to convince animals to sleep through the winter. And what is the purpose of fat? To get animals through lean times of extreme famine when they need to restrict movement and lay around doing as little as possible. Fat exists to prepare for hibernation and fat punishes those behaving otherwise.

You need not be fat. You need not spend your life being punished by your body.

"...open up and drink in all that white light, pouring down from the heaven, haven't got time for the pain"

— Carly Simon

Regaining Health Step By Step: an Antidote to Your Poisoned Plate

"You are what you eat - so don't be cheap, fast, easy or fake" —American Proverb

"At heart we are all powerful, beautiful, and capable of changing the world with our bare hands."
— Dianne Sylvan, *The Body Sacred*

As my patients and students can attest, if you make it through my lectures, you do leave with specific advice. Your task is finding which of these advisements you can sustain. People are different — and temporary changes will not result in a healthy body.

Eating correctly is currently more expensive and time-consuming. However, if roughly 18% of American consumers took the steps that follow, the profit margins of conventional products would fall enough to force change in massive food farms and corporations, making the less toxic alternatives relatively more affordable.

Many of my patients have found gradual changes easier to accommodate in their daily lives. To that end, a practical guide to Your Poisoned Plates is being reviewed. For now, here is an effective antidote to your poison plate:

Eliminate all processed meats.

Work toward eliminating all animal flesh except birds and fish from your diet.

Increase your fruits and vegetables to at least 5 servings a day.

Incorporate healthy oils into your diet.

Eliminate anything in a box or prepacked bag unless it is loose-frozen and only has one ingredient.

Choose local produce whenever possible.

Eliminate all wheat, grains and all but wild (black) rice or ancient grains from your diet.

Choose organic produce. Choose only organic dairy products and only pasture-fed organic or wild-caught animals.

Reduce alcohol to less than 1 measured drink daily.

Do not smoke (anything).

Eat more raw foods; do not charbroil anything.

Avoid eating anything with a label on it. If it needs a label and has more than three ingredients, it is probably toxic.

Drink pure water with every meal and at least twice between meals.

Do not eat anything you cannot pronounce and that doesn't grow on a farm, forest or in the lake/ocean in the form you are eating it.

Incorporate naturally fermented products with biologically active cultures into your diet, such as yoghurt, kefir, miso, raw apple cider vinegar, sauerkraut and kimchee. These help maintain your microbiome.

Monthly after bathing, rinse your hair and skin with a mixture of 4 ounces each kefir and yoghurt and a tablespoon of raw apple cider vinegar. (Avoid eyes or it will sting). Rinse and pat dry.

Enjoy spices made from organic plants; start your own organic herbs.

Garden: Get your hands dirty and occasionally go barefoot.

Reduce the man-made chemicals in your home.

Reduce your exposure to fluoride. Use dental floss not mouthwash. Use toothpaste without fluoride. See your dental hygienist regularly even if you don't have insurance but skip the routine xrays. If you are prone to cavities in your permanent teeth, your dentist can apply specific fluoride gel or seal your molar crevices.

Canned food has BPA and BPA liners. Don't buy canned food (not even soup).

Plastic bottles labeled with a recycled triangle Δ and a "1" or "2" in the triangle do not have BPA. Most single serving bottled water is "1"; most canned water has BPA. Glass and metal are safer, but if you use plastic adhere to the above and never put plastic bottles in the microwave.

Don't put anything in or on your vagina, rectum, skin or hair that you wouldn't eat.

Never use antiperspirant. Consider deodorant with natural ingredients only — the vagina rule applies (see above).

Reduce your exposure to dry cleaning chemicals. Stop using fabric softener in any form. Use bleach on clothing only for spot stains.

Eliminate all antibiotics and antifungal in any form from your home. This includes all antibacterial soaps.

Always ask your doctor if you can get better without antibiotics. 90% of infections are either *not* bacterial (antibiotics are useless against virus infections) or can be cleared by helping your body drain the infection. Never ask for antibiotics and never self-treat with antibiotics from someone else or from an old prescription.

Eliminate herbicides, pesticides and fungicides in or around your home and air your home out twice a month (more during months you are heating). Bathrooms and kitchens should be aired more frequently. No kitchen or bathroom should vent back into the house — fix it.

Sleep more. Adults who sleep eight hours a night are thinner than adults who sleep less.

Do you not know that you are God's temple and that God's Spirit dwells in you? If anyone destroys God's temple, God will destroy him. For God's temple is holy, and you are that temple. —1 Corinthians 3:16 - 17. The Bible

You Have But One Life — Rise Up And Live It.

Appendix

Actionable Resources toward Detoxification

Where do you find what you need to avoid poisoning yourself? Here are some resources to begin a healthier life. You will have to determine which products will help bring you health as some company products may not align with detoxification even though other products do.

Fermentation, Composting and Canning
Lehman's
289 Kurzen Road
N. Dalton OH 44618
Lehmans.com

Organic Herbs and Spices
Frontier Natural Products Co-op
PO Box 299
3021 78th St.
Norway, IA 52318
frontiercoop.com

Pest Management
American Natural Products
2103 185th Street
Fairfield IA 52556
Americanatural.com

Gardens, Lawns and Pests
Gardens Alive!
5100 Schenley Place
Lawrenceburg IN 47025
gardensalive.com

Fragrances and Essential Oils
NOW
244 Knollwood Drive, Suite 300
Bloomingdale, IL 60108
nowfoods.com

Soaps and Cleaners
Seventh Generation
60 Lake Street
Burlington, VT 05401
seventhgeneration.com

Dental Care (some fluoride-free products)

Tom's of Maine
Consumer Dialogue Department
302 Lafayette Center
Kennebunk, ME 04043

tomsofmaine.com